NOT ALWAYS
A VALLEY
OF TEARS

A Memoir of a Life Well Lived

PASCUALA HERRERA

This is a memoir. Some names have been changed; some events have been compressed; and some dialogue has been re-created.

To view personal photos and more, please visit Pascuala online at pascualaherrera.com.

Cover design: 100 Covers
Interior design: Formatted Books
Copy editor: Allison Felus

Printed in the United States of America

To my parents,
Eulalio and Virginia Herrera,
who sacrificed everything for our family;
my brothers, sisters, and their families;

and above all,
my loving family,
Isidro, Ariel, and Ariana

ACKNOWLEDGMENTS

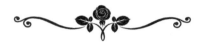

I have so many people to thank. Some have left this world to be in a better place, like my parents. My dad and mom have always been my heroes. They made so many sacrifices for each of their children, but especially for me. I am especially grateful to my mom who never gave up on me and who always kept the faith even when no one else had it. She was my rod to lean on, the one that I counted on for everything. My mom was gentle and loving, but tough and stern when she needed to be. She pushed me to be all that I could be even when it tore her apart. My dad lived for his family and did all he could to make sure we had the best of this life. I am here because of them. I owe them every success and every accomplishment. I still remember all the stories they shared and have used many of these stories to recount what happened in my early years since I didn't have many memories of my childhood. I have tried to retell the many stories as accurately as possible. Sometimes, the names I use are fictitious to protect a person's identity, but the events are real, viewed from my perspective and memory.

I also thank each member of my family, especially my brothers and sisters, for always accepting me and looking out for what was best for me. Thank you for helping me fill in the holes to the beginning of my life.

In addition, I have always been blessed with having the best friends ever because they have supported, encouraged, and cared for me each step of the way. In each stage of my life, I have met the most wonderful people, many who became friends for life.

And of course, I am eternally thankful for my husband, Isidro, and two beautiful daughters, Ariel and Ariana, who completed me. Without them, I wouldn't be the successful, fulfilled woman that I am today.

I am also appreciative of everyone who supported the publishing of this book. I thank Maria Sotelo and Gerardo Alanis, two friends who encouraged me and became my support throughout this unfamiliar process. Of course, I could not have published without the professional support from my copy editor, Allison Felus.

Above all, I am thankful to God. Because of his loving grace, all things were possible.

PREFACE

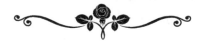

Now that I am over half a century old and have accomplished so many things that seemed impossible, I am taking the time to relive many experiences, the good and the difficult. Most people will never understand how it is that my mind is full of energy, yet my body does not want to follow. In my mind, I am still that young, risk-taking girl who always realized she was different but never let it stop her from pushing forward. Now my body constantly reminds me that those days are over. Those who have known me all my life cannot accept this change and say that I am still too young to have such an attitude and that it must be some sort of depression. However, I am fully at peace with this change and just need to help those around me realize that this "new me" is not a worse me. This new me is not giving up, nor is she in some sort of depression. It is quite simple. This new me just wants to rest.

I'm at the top of the mountain. I look across the horizon and take a deep breath as I savor the realization that I made it to the top. I made it! I am living what I dreamed of. I am living my utopia. So, as I look all around me, I look deep in my soul and question, "Am I happy?" The answer does not come out quickly and spontaneously as it should. I analyze all that I have, and all that I've accomplished, and rationally tell myself that I am happy. But happiness does not come from the mind, it comes from the heart. And, happiness has no rational stance. For if it were rational, then it would be apparent that I am happy, for I have accomplished each goal that I have put forward. The heart is more complicated! It's not a formula that you can put together. Sometimes it won't add up. Like in my case! My heart is heavy, though it should be light with happiness.

As long as I can remember, this heaviness in my heart has been there. I never perceived this weight as bad, for it always served me well and made me get to the next step in my life. That which weighed down my heart lifted my soul. I so much wanted to make my heart lighter and happier that I immediately immersed myself in the next project, the next goal, the next deadline, the next success. It numbed me. Although the heaviness was there, it energized me to move forward and carry on. No one in my surroundings noticed the heaviness of my heart. All they saw were my accomplishments. They saw me as happy—superhuman even—certainly stronger than any obstacle in front of her. I fooled them.

Now, though, I am letting the heaviness of my heart set in. It is a scary feeling, for never did I take the time to be in touch with those feelings. However, in my mind, and even in a tiny corner of my heart, I think that this will be yet my greatest accomplishment. I will be able to finally recognize what is in my heart, set all my burdens down, and perhaps empty some of that weight into the abyss for me never to feel again.

The process is not easy, for as humans we are conditioned by routine. I must shift paradigms and the shift will be a total twist. I am sure that many tears, many fears, and many unwanted issues will surface. But I am equally sure that once at the surface, I will conquer that which is in me. I will rise to the top. It is perhaps through this reflection that I will understand that, though my life has been difficult, it's not always a valley of tears. Sometimes, the tears themselves have grown the most beautiful rose gardens.

CHAPTER 1

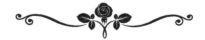

I often have said that my mom gave me life twice. The first time was when she carried me in her womb to full term, and the second time was about a year and a half after I was born when her love and faith brought me back to life. I honestly think God's grace chose my mom, who was justly named Virginia, to give me life two times. Like Virgin Mary, she was entrusted with a very difficult responsibility—caring for me and helping me live a purposeful and productive life.

My life hasn't been easy, but it has been marvelous! I was born on May 17, 1965. The eighth child of a family of nine, I was born in the small town of La Purísima (which translates as "The Purest"), by a midwife who had also delivered my siblings.

La Purísima is a small town on the outskirts of Tepehuanes in Durango, Mexico. There are approximately two hundred and fifty inhabitants, all connected to each other in some way or another. The homes in the town had no running water or electricity at that time. The nearest source of water, a couple of miles away, was a stream with the most beautiful cascade. The town only had one school, which was about a mile from most homes. There was no hospital or medical care except for the unofficial nurse who healed by means of home remedies and, on occasion, would inject people with medicine she brought from Tepehuanes.

To most people this would resemble a third-world country stricken with the utmost poverty, but to the inhabitants, La Purísima was a piece of heaven on earth. Everyone knew everyone. Kids played freely in the streets amongst the stray pigs and animals. It was normal to hear the oinking of pigs being bothered by the children. Each morning, the alarm clock was the crowing of a rooster beginning his busy day at the crack of dawn.

The men, when they were wealthy enough to have their own farm and animals, were responsible for farming and taking care of the livestock. Otherwise, it was not unheard of for them to go to the United States, often undocumented, to earn money to support their families. This was the case for my dad, Eulalio. He immigrated to the United States in 1956, six years after marrying my mom.

My mom was only seventeen and my dad was twenty-five when they got married, though their first interaction was when my mom was about eight years old and my dad sixteen. My dad was spinning a handmade top while my mom watched. My dad, being a rambunctious teenager, thought it would be fun to pick up the spinning top and place it on my mom's head. Of course, it was only funny until he saw how painfully the top wound my mom's hair into a tight knot. My mom ran to her mother crying while the top still dangled from her head. My grandmother, whom we called Mama Petra, was *not* happy. She scolded my dad and complained to his mother, Tina (whom we later called Mama Tina). Of course, at that time, no one would have imagined that my dad would make my mom his wife on September 15, 1950. My parents told me this story many times, and every time, I would smile, imagining my mom's beautiful brown hair all tangled up while my dad was trying to hide under a rock.

Although my dad's family was more well-off compared to my mom's family, my dad had been a free spirit who never settled down. He was known to just hang out and drink with friends when he was not in the fields helping his parents. He never attended even one day of school. When he got married, it was the first time he wore a pair of shoes, not just because they didn't have much money but also because he didn't like them. My grandparents were strict, however, and demanded that my dad be responsible and take care of his family. They were strong Catholics and demanded good values and behavior. My dad always felt that he never met his parents' expectations, often telling me stories of how he disappointed his father.

My dad told me a story that I will never forget. Once when he was already a grown man but still single, he was out on the farm. One of the cattle had strayed to someone else's property so he went to get it. He noticed a few apples on the ground that had fallen from an apple tree. Without much thought, he grabbed one and began to eat it. My grandfather had followed him, though, and saw my dad beginning to eat the apple. He approached him and asked, "Is this land yours?" My dad replied, "No," still not knowing where the conversation was heading. My grandfather, still on his horse, then asked, "Is this apple tree yours?" Again, my dad responded, "No." He asked a third question, "Are those apples yours?" pointing down to the apples. My dad for the third time said "No." My grandfather was quiet for a few seconds, then got off his horse and asked, "Did someone give you those apples?" My dad looked down, and this time just nodded no. Without saying anything, my grandfather took off his belt and whipped him good. When he was done, my grandfather said, "Never take anything that doesn't belong to you." When my dad recounted this story, my heart hurt for him. I wanted so badly to defend my dad. I admired him so much, especially because he told me the story without any resentment, but instead wanted to teach me a lesson that he had learned.

Without an education, my dad's only way to support his family was to earn money in the United States. He decided to cross over illegally, just six years after marrying my mom. It was a decision they made together because it was the only way they could survive, especially now that they had three daughters with another on the way. I can't imagine the fear both my dad and mom felt as they faced the unknown.

He saved some money to pay a coyote. Coyotes were usually US citizens who charged undocumented Mexicans to help them cross the border, usually through inhumane conditions. All my dad took with him were the clothes on his back, but he was willing to take the risk for a better life for his family. My dad visited home every other year because he couldn't stay away too long from his family. And with each visit, the family got bigger! Sometimes immigration would catch him and bring him back to Mexico, but he would just turn around and try to cross again. Immigration was much easier at the time, so he became a legal resident of the US a few years later. It was so eye-opening for me to learn about how dangerous it was to cross over into the United States while undocumented. But it was obvious that his hope for a better life was always greater than any fear he felt.

My mom came from a poor family and was the oldest female of six siblings. Her mother, Mama Petra, became widowed early in life, so my mom practically raised her younger siblings. My mom had only attended a few years of school by the time she had to quit to help her family. My mom's essence was to be a servant since that was what she learned early on in her life. She was one of the most hardworking women I'd ever met, always putting everyone's needs before her own. She was full of virtues, but what made her even more wonderful was that she never saw her own most wonderful qualities. Her humbleness made her shine, giving life to all she touched. Her legacy was to care for her siblings, children, grandchildren, and any living plant she touched. Her legacy lives in all of us.

My mom once told me a story that really put into perspective the extent of her poverty. When she was a teenager, her family could hardly afford to put food on the table, so she definitely didn't have money to buy makeup. But she smiled when she shared how she figured out a way to fit in. She said, "I couldn't buy makeup, so I decided to make my own. I wanted to have rosy cheeks, so I grabbed a reddish-brown brick and scraped it. I collected the dust and rubbed it on my cheeks." Of course, she didn't need makeup since she was naturally beautiful, which I'm glad my dad recognized.

In La Purísima, women were responsible for the home and care of the children, though older children quickly took on the responsibility of helping with their younger siblings. Several times a week, women would walk to a stream with jugs on their heads to fetch water or would stay there even longer to wash clothing. My mom couldn't afford store-bought clothes, so what money my dad was able to send was either used to buy food or to buy fabric to make clothes. Women learned how to stretch the money they received, buying sacks of beans and rice that could last for a long time. Seafood was unheard of, and meat was only prepared on very special occasions when it could be shared with extended family.

I have always enjoyed having a big family, though I might feel differently if I had been one of the oldest. Being the baby girl had many perks. Still, I have no idea how my parents, with such a lack of resources, managed to feed and clothe us all. Regardless, all of us adopted the strong values that my parents instilled in us.

Our family consists of six girls and three boys. My parents would take turns deciding the name of each child, and the names my dad chose were always peculiar. Interestingly, he decided to name me Pascuala, after St. Paschal Baylón, who had died on the date of my birth, May 17, in 1592.

During his life St. Paschal Baylón was known as a saint who was always happy, cheerful, full of life, and respectful of everyone. Only many years later did my parents discover the significance of my being named after him and knew that it was not a coincidence but all part of God's divine plan. When I was younger, I hated my name, just because many people found it hard to pronounce and to spell. But as an adult, I came to like my name for its uniqueness and especially for being named after a saint.

The names of the rest of my family members, in birth order, along with our nicknames are

Eulalio Herrera	February 12, 1925
Virginia Diaz	August 15, 1933
Silveria "Bella"	June 20, 1951

Maria de los Angeles "Angelita"	May 31, 1953
Teresa "Tere"	March 11, 1955
Francisca "Kika"	April 3, 1957
Jose Ramon "Mon"	May 20, 1960
Reynalda "Reyna"	October 29, 1961
Eulalio Jr. "Lalo"	May 9, 1963
Pascuala "Cuali"	May 17, 1965
Enrique "Rique"	February 21, 1967

We were poor, and because my dad only visited the family every two years, the bulk of the responsibility for the day-to-day care of the family fell on my mom's shoulders. I cannot imagine the pressure my mom must have felt in raising all of us without the presence of my dad. My older sisters helped with my care when my mom was busy doing other chores.

I was born healthy and without any noteworthy issues. In fact, my first several months of life were uneventful except for my eagerness to walk. By the age of nine months, I was already walking, hanging on to furniture.

One morning that winter, my paternal grandparents had slaughtered a pig and brought some meat to our home. My mom hurried around the house doing a multitude of chores, including preparing the pork to cook. In the rush of the day, my mom kept an eye out as my oldest sisters, who were fourteen and twelve at the time, watched me. As she cut up the pork with the only dull knife she had, she put the pieces on a piece of twine hung across the kitchen as if she was hanging clothes to dry. Several times, my mom yelled out, "Estan bien?" wanting assurance that I was doing okay. My sisters were just happy that I was not giving them much trouble. But when it came time for my mom to feed me, she picked me up from where they had put me and noticed that I had a high fever. Immediately she wet a cloth with cool water from the jarro (jug) to put on my fore-head. My mom had to rely on home remedies because we didn't even have enough money for an aspirin in the house. She asked my sisters, "Didn't you notice she was hot? Why didn't you come and get me?"

My mom became concerned when my fever didn't go down. She felt my body go limp and my eyes were barely open. She waited for a while, continuing with the cold compresses, but I seemed to be getting worse. She instructed my sisters to stay home and watch the rest of the kids because she was going to take me to see the local nurse with the hope of getting some type of medication to bring my fever down. She wrapped me in a blanket and walked, almost in a trot, down several streets to the nurse's house. The nurse quickly laid me on a bed to examine me. She became alarmed and said, "I cannot help. She needs a doctor, and she needs to see one quick!" My mom wrapped me up again and rushed me to my dad's parents' house to ask for help, since no one in her own family had a vehicle. Tepehuanes is about two hours away, and she needed someone to take me since the buses had stopped running already. My uncle Gabriel, one of my dad's younger brothers, was there, and he quickly volunteered to drive us to Tepehuanes. My mom told my uncle Gabriel that she had only a few pesos, but my uncle told her not to worry, as he quickly looked in his wallet.

We got in the back seat of his truck and stopped briefly by my house to tell my sisters to get everyone in bed since it was almost 10 PM. My mom instructed my sisters, "Watch your brothers and sisters. I don't know how long I will be gone." My sisters, both with startled faces, nodded yes. My mom then directed them, "Go get Mama Petra so you're not alone." My mom tightly held me, and by this time, I was unresponsive. As my sister Bella was putting on her sweater to go get Mama Petra, my mom pleaded, "Gabriel, let's hurry, please."

The road to Tepehuanes is very rocky, and with each bump, my mom held me tighter. Many cars often slid off the road, especially in the rain or if it was dark. And sure enough, my uncle lost control during one of the turns, and the truck went down into a ditch.

Fortunately, we were strapped in, and my mom had such a tight grip on me that no one got hurt. My uncle tried every way he could to get us out, but he was unsuccessful. He told my mom, "Comadre, I am going to go get help. There is a gas station up ahead." My mom, still startled, asked, "How far is it?" He responded, "I will walk about three miles to get help." My mom tried to be strong but began to cry. My uncle reassured her, "I will come back as quickly as I can." Often, when my mom told me this story, she would become agitated, as if she relived the trauma of such a nerve-wracking experience.

My mom was in the back seat in pitch darkness rocking me back and forth. In her anguish she prayed nonstop. Unsure of the time, my mom felt it was an eternity by the time my uncle came with someone in a truck to pull us out. My uncle paid the man who pulled us out, and as soon as the truck was out the ditch, we quickly continued our way.

By this time, my uncle had decided to take me straight to the city of Durango instead of to Tepehuanes. Tepehuanes didn't have a hospital and the clinic was already closed since it was close to 2:00 AM. Durango is another two-hour drive from Tepehuanes, but my uncle tried to calm my mom down by explaining to her that at least the roads would be much better. At about 4 AM, my uncle arrived at the main hospital. He helped my mom out as she continued to hold me tight. We were greeted by a nurse, and as she led us to an examining room, my mom urged her, "Hurry, she is not moving."

My mom noticed that the nurse put on a mask and gloves and never touched my frail body. She instructed my mom and uncle to lay me on the bed and to loosen me from all the blankets my mom had me wrapped in. She said, "Let me go get the doctor," and quickly turned away. As she was leaving, my mom implored with a begging voice, "Please hurry."

Within a minute, Doctor Medina came into the room. Before even introducing himself, he put on a protective mask and gloves. He then started to speak as he began examining me. "In the United States, I have heard there is a big epidemic of a serious disease." Before he named the disease, he started asking a series of questions one after another, without even waiting for a response. "Is anyone else sick in the home? How long has she been like this? Did you give her anything to eat or drink? Did you give her any medicine?"

Dr. Medina listened to my heart and my lungs and said, "It's good, she is breathing." He opened my eyelids with a finger and with a bright flashlight examined the reaction of my pupils. He just shook his head. He squeezed my toes, my legs, my fingers, and my arms to see if I would react. Again, he just shook his head while scratching it, saying, "Esto es serio."

My mom picked me up and held me again in her arms and asked, "Doctor what can you do?" He said, "There is a bad disease that is killing many people in the United States and all over the world. It is called poliomyelitis. This child has polio." My mom had never heard such a word, but she knew it was bad because of the doctor's tone. The doctor went on to say, "There is nothing to do. She will likely die any minute." Dr. Medina continued, "Any minute, she will stop breathing, just like she stopped moving. There is nothing to do. Just prepare for her death."

The doctor then left the room. My uncle embraced my mom with me still in her arms and tried to console her. How do you console a mom whose hope was just shattered? She cried for what seemed an eternity, until her sobs were interrupted by a crew of several doctors and nurses. As I learned about what the doctor said, I admired my mom so much more, for not breaking down and giving up. This would be what most women in her situation would have done.

My mom stopped crying and, for a moment, when she saw the group of doctors and nurses, she had a new surge of hope. Maybe there was something that could be done. Maybe the doctors came to wake me up and cure me. Dr. Medina grabbed me from my mom's arms without asking or saying a word. He lay me on the table and began poking and prodding me, demonstrating to everyone that I was almost lifeless. The doctor said, "Polio means death." He then sat down on a chair and started to talk to my mom and uncle. He said,

"I am sorry, but your daughter has a very serious disease, and it is very contagious." My mom almost fell to the ground, but he continued, "You must wear a mask and not hold her so close to you. Also, we need to keep her in a separate room until she dies to make sure polio does not spread."

My mom looked at my uncle, and then the doctor, wanting them to say it was a mistake. As the doctor took off his gloves and washed his hands, he said "As soon as we can, we will call the Red Cross to come and help us to make sure no one else in your town gets this disease. Listen very clearly; this is very dangerous." My mom always remembered the words that Dr. Medina said. With tears in her eyes, she would relive that awful moment, the doctor's words echoing in her mind over fifty years later.

In Durango, the mornings are always twenty degrees colder, and especially in February, the temperatures can drop down to the fifties. My mom was saddened to see the sun rising because this meant that this was not just a bad dream she was having. Indeed, this was reality. She watched as phone calls were made, and nurses and doctors ran around with their masks and gloves on. One of the nurses offered my mom a cup of coffee, but my mom didn't even look up. She still held me, even against the doctor's advice. The nurse reminded my mom, "Put on your mask." But again, my mom didn't respond and just looked down at me.

Later that morning, I was escorted with my mom to a hospital room. My uncle had filled out the paperwork, and though my mom didn't have any money, my uncle signed on her behalf. The hospital room was very simple, but what my mom remembered most was a big crucifix hanging on the wall above the bed. She immediately was mesmerized by it and began to pray endlessly. She kept saying over and over, "God, please don't take her." My uncle told my mom "I have to go back to La Purísima, but I will be back." My mom urged him, "Please check on all my kids." He promised he would. He then put an arm around her and said, "Comadre, entregela a Dios (give her to God).” My mom screamed back at him and yelled “Never! I will never return her back to God!”

The entire day, my mom just held my lifeless body. She kept checking to ensure that I was still breathing. Night fell and my mom still prayed. When morning came, my uncle arrived back. He told my mom, “We can go home now.” My mom said, “But they haven’t done anything for her. She is still not moving.” My uncle said, “There is nothing they can do. There is no use staying in the hospital when they won’t do anything.” He looked at me and asked, “Esta mejor?” Sadly, my mom nodded and acknowledged that I wasn’t better as tears started flowing again. My uncle said, “The Red Cross went to La Purísima and vaccinated everyone. It is safe to return home.” He explained, “The rest of the family is now vaccinated, so it is safe now because they have the polio vaccine.” My mom had not had a bite to eat for over twenty-four hours, so my uncle offered her a piece of bread. She ate it without much enthusiasm as she listened to all the Red Cross commotion that she had missed while she held me the whole previous day. Why I was the only one to get polio, we will never know. All my other seven brothers and sisters never had any sign of it, although my brothers did have febrile seizures when they were infants but recuperated as they grew. This diagnosis changed not only my life but the lives of everyone in my family.

CHAPTER 2

With disillusioned hearts, my mom and uncle left the hospital and began the travel back to La Purísima. There was no conversation, each lost in their own thoughts. My mom was searching for an explanation of why I contracted polio. She was retracing everything that had happened the previous few days. She asked herself, "Was it something I did? Was it something my daughters fed her? Did she come in contact with something harmful? Why was she the one with this bad disease?" The questions just raced in her head. The more she thought, the more she looked for blame and an explanation.

Along with these thoughts, she began to feel guilt and wished she hadn't been so busy the day before. She hated that she had not protected me from whatever caused me to get this disease. She wondered if the pork my grandparents gave her was contaminated. She tried to remember if I had touched or been too close to the meat hanging in the kitchen. My mom started to feel more and more anxious. Even with this anxiety, she refused to accept that I would die even though Dr. Medina had stressed that I would most likely stop breathing. She looked down at me and couldn't help the tears that filled her eyes.

Other thoughts came to her that filled her with despair. My uncle had paid the hospital costs and she knew it had been expensive even though the hospital didn't do anything. All the hospital did was to diagnose me with that awful disease that had affected so many people the previous decade. She recalled Dr. Medina's explanation over and over. Dr. Medina explained that the disease spread everywhere, including the United States. He told her that a vaccine had been developed in the States, but that Mexico was just hearing about it. He explained why it had been important to vaccinate everyone in the town. He also insisted on vaccinating my mom, though my mom couldn't worry about anything other than the baby she was holding.

My uncle had his own thoughts but didn't share much during the trip. He kept looking back, checking to see if my mom's expression of sorrow had changed. After a couple of hours, he suggested they stop in Tepehuanes and insisted that my mom try to reach my dad so that he could be informed. He paid so that my mom could make a long-distance call. Because it was early afternoon, she didn't know if my dad would be available.

At the time, my dad was living in Chicago, working in a factory. He got this opportunity after working for several years in California, picking strawberries for five cents an hour. My dad decided to move to Chicago and started operating punch-press machinery for twenty-five cents an hour. My uncle knew the factory's phone number because he had two other brothers who also worked there. He dialed the number, and my mom was almost wishing that they wouldn't be able to reach him because she had no idea how she would share such devastating news.

My uncle asked for my dad and when he was told they would get him, he handed my mom the phone. After a couple of minutes of silence, my dad came on the phone. My mom mumbled a couple of words and then was no longer able to speak as she saw me in her arms still lifeless. My uncle took the phone, saying "Brother, your daughter Pascualita is very sick and the doctors don't give much hope." My dad was asking lots of questions, but my uncle was not able to respond to many. He hung up the phone and walked us back to the truck.

A couple of hours later, we arrived at our house. The cement house was painted in bright blue. As my uncle pulled up in front, the two wooden front doors opened wide. Mama Petra came out holding my brother Lalo who was not even three years old. After her, all other six siblings came out to greet us, as if we were arriving with treats. My mom's sunken eyes were all that Mama Petra had to see to know that things were not good. My uncle helped my mom climb the high curb in front of our house and guided her inside. He gave Mama Petra a brief greeting and update, and then left. My mom thanked him as he walked out.

My mom sat down on the bed, still holding me. She tried to smile as she looked around at the other seven kids around her. Mama Petra suggested she rest and told her to lay me down. My mom was tired, but she also couldn't think of resting. Mama Petra asked to hold me and started to rock me. She mimicked talking to me and telling me to not be lazy and wake up. She noticed that I felt heavy because I was motionless. Mama Petra tried to console my mom, and said, "Hija, God is calling her back home and you have to accept His will." My mom responded back saying, "No; she is not going to die. She will wake up." Mama Petra insisted one more time by saying, "She is God's child and you have to be strong and accept that she is going to die." Instead of being consoled, my mom raised her voice and told Mama Petra, "I don't want to hear that she is going to die, so stop!!" All my brothers and sisters quieted down when they heard my mom's voice raised. Mama Petra handed me back to my mom and pushed the little ones out to play. My older sisters asked my mom if she wanted some rice that Mama Petra had cooked. With a shake of her head, my mom said no.

When nightfall came, Mama Petra went home. My mom held me as she got everyone off to bed. The house we lived in had a total of four rooms (a front room, two bedrooms, and a kitchen) and an outhouse in the fenced corral. All the rooms, except the kitchen, were used for sleeping. My five sisters slept in two beds in one of the bedrooms. My mom and I slept in one bed and my two brothers in another bed in the second bedroom. The front room also had a bed so Mama Petra or other visitors could sleep. The evenings tended to be cool, so my mom ensured we had plenty of warm blankets to cover us.

My mom was the last one to get to bed. She was exhausted after carrying me all day. She didn't want to lay me down and possibly miss some sign of life. Her faith was amazing. She was even afraid to go to sleep in fear of missing some movement from me. She decided to make a cradle using her legs wrapped tightly in a blanket, to lay me down as she slept. She figured that by having me sleep on her legs, she would feel me moving. Tiredness got the better of her, and she finally dozed off.

After a few hours of sleep, my mom was roused by the wake-up call from the rooster. Though we didn't have cows, horses, or pigs, we did have chickens in the corral. In addition, the corral had two huge prickly pears trees, nopales. The morning routine consisted of her going to gather the eggs and collect any ripe prickly pears, tunas. However, this morning it was different.

Due to my illness, she had to establish a different routine. She was disappointed to see that I had not moved all night. I was still swaddled in the same position she had left me at night. Her new routine was to first check on me to make sure I was still breathing. She placed her hand near my nose and mouth to feel my breath. Next, using her hands, she lightly opened my eyes. Additionally, she noticed my feet were always freezing cold. Using her warm breath, she would blow on them and rub them until they got warm. My mom's love was so strong. She clung to me and didn't let me go. She wanted her love to be my medicine and lived as if I would always be a part of her life.

Another step to the new routine was to somehow nourish me. At the hospital, I had received IV fluids, but at home, my mom was unsure how to feed me. Just days before, I would be nourished with breast milk and had just begun eating soft foods. Now, my mom knew that breastfeeding wouldn't work. The only solution she found was to drop milk in my mouth with a spoon. She had to learn the best pace. She was startled when she dropped several spoonsful of milk and I appeared to be choking. She had to raise my head so that the milk would slide down my throat.

This new way of feeding me took time. She would manage to give me several ounces of milk each morning, taking her an hour to do so. Her dedicated love probably nourished me more than the several spoonfuls of milk she managed to feed me. My older three sisters, aged fourteen, twelve, and ten, had to step up and do more to help my mom. They got the eggs and cooked breakfast to ensure that the school-aged kids got ready to walk to school. My brother, Lalo, who was about to be three stayed with my mom and me.

Other parts of the day's routines had to change as well. My mom became unsure if she could take my brother and me to the stream as she normally did before my illness. She worried that something bad would happen and felt it important to always keep an eye on me, always praying that I would show some type of movement. She always kept her faith even after days, weeks, and months passed by. She held me and talked to me as if I could listen to her. "Mija, despierta. It's time to wake up. You can't leave me!" She told me about all that I was missing: "Look how beautiful today is. The sun is shining." She prayed out loud, "Dios, please have pity on me. I know she is yours, but I need her." She bargained with God, "I promise that I will always be with her and care for her if you let her live."

Three months after my illness, in May, around my first birthday, my dad came back early for his vacation from work in Chicago. Usually, he would come in August, but due to my condition, he took his vacation as soon as he could. When he entered our home, everyone greeted him, though my five-year-old sister, Reyna, and my three-year-old brother, Lalo, didn't remember him and were intimidated, hiding behind my mom who was holding me. After he hugged each of my siblings, he hugged my mom with me in between. He looked down, and he was surprised that I looked so peaceful and appeared to be sleeping.

While in Chicago, after talking to my uncle Gabriel on the phone, he had imagined me differently. He took me from my mom's arms and held me as he proceeded to sit on an old wooden chair. He looked at me intensely, as a couple of tears rolled down his cheeks.

He began asking my mom questions about my progress and was disappointed to hear that there had been no change in my condition in the previous three months. My dad held my little arm and raised it without resistance and noticed how it just dropped when he let it go. He kissed me on the forehead and held me a bit tighter. My mom heard him mumble when he said he was sorry.

As usual, my dad was only going to be home on vacation for two weeks and then would be returning to Chicago. He had gotten his green card, though, so at least he didn't have to risk getting caught each time he came to see the family. He brought each of his children a new outfit, imagining the sizes based on the previous visit. He also brought simple toys and candy. The family felt that his visits were the real Christmas because of all the gifts he brought. He tried as much as possible to learn what he had missed in the previous two years. At night, my mom and dad would talk for hours catching up. Though now he felt that he had to work harder than ever to pay my uncle back for the hospital costs.

As he observed what my mom did for me each day and how she dressed me, fed me, and took care of me with such devotion, my dad felt heart broken. Although he never verbalized it, he worried about my mom and whether she was going to be prepared for me dying. On the other hand, my mom's faith was contagious, and like my mom, my dad clung to hope. He felt that I was still alive for some reason and prayed that I would wake up at any time. One night, my mom fell asleep with me between her legs with the blanket she used as a cradle, and my dad contemplated the sight and began to speak to God asking, "Dios, please let her live. I promise I will always be here and will always provide for her and all my family."

Two weeks passed and my dad had to return to Chicago. Although it was always a sad moment each time he had to leave, this time it was even more difficult for my parents to say goodbye. They hugged each other tightly. My dad promised to send more money and told my mom he loved her. He turned around and tearfully walked out the door. My mom, who never allowed her children to see her cry, quickly started to direct the children to their chores or to play. She tried to sound cheerful though she was distraught. She had felt supported during my dad's visit, but now that she was all alone again. She had no one else to help her deal with the pain of seeing me motionless.

CHAPTER 3

Weeks after my dad had left, my mom received her miracle. She couldn't believe what she was seeing. She noticed that I moved my head from side to side. At first, it was slow and rare. But as time went on, I moved my head side to side more often. She was ecstatic. Though others were happy for this change, they felt obligated to remind my mom that my future didn't look promising. My mom was beginning to get used to this type of commentary. In the beginning, she would get angry, but eventually, she simply learned to ignore it.

This head movement made my mom happier than she had been in a long time. She was so happy that she had to go to Tepehuanes to call Chicago to let my dad know. She left my siblings with Mama Petra and took me on the bus to Tepehuanes to make such an important call. Her voice was radiating as she told my dad about my improvement. She talked about it as if I had accomplished the greatest feat. With pride she shared, "She keeps moving her head." She giggled as she explained, "I have to be careful when I feed her because I might get the blended food all over her clothes." She smiled and my dad felt it through the phone. After the call, she went to buy some fabric since she needed to make some new clothes because we were all growing too fast. She also bought a box of cookies and a bottle of Pepsi. She got this treat for the family on special occasions and she felt that this merited a celebration. After shopping, she took the bus back to

La Purísima and for the whole two-hour trip she smiled. It had been a good day. She thanked God nonstop all the way home, "Gracias, Dios mío, gracias."

My mom received another sign that her prayers were being answered. She divided the box of cookies among each of her kids. Her distribution was based on age. The older the child, the more cookies each would get. She was so happy that she decided to include me in the distribution for the first time. She grabbed one cookie and soaked it with Pepsi, crushing it with a spoon until it was like a paste. She put some in my mouth and that is when she noticed that I moved my right pinky finger. She thought she was seeing visions, but when she fed me another spoonful, I moved the pinky again. Again, to her, this movement was as if I had won a gold medal in the Olympics. It is no wonder that one of my mom's favorite sayings was, "Mientras haya vida, hay esperanza. (As long as there is life, there is hope.)"

It had been six months since my polio diagnosis, and by this time, I was now able to move my head, open my eyes, and moved my right arm. My recovery was ever so gradual, but my mom waited patiently. My mom was filled with joy. Around this time, she also learned that she was pregnant for the ninth time. My dad's visit had left her pregnant, which explained why each child was born approximately two years apart with several being born in May due to my dad's usual vacation in August. My mom was never disappointed to be pregnant even with her struggles financially. Likewise, my dad was filled with joy each time he learned about each of us. My dad regularly expressed how he was the richest man in the world due to his sons and daughters.

My mom was so thankful that I was starting to react and thanked God for bringing me back to life and for the new life that was growing in her womb. As her pregnancy started to show, I was likewise starting to show more signs of improvement. Each new movement was a milestone that brought my mom even more hope. I started moving my arms, and my babbling was like music to her ears. She did notice that I had not moved my legs, but she was content with me waking up on my own. My mom encouraged me to move more. She was convinced that a cookie and Pepsi would motivate me to move my arm to feed myself. She screamed for joy as I grabbed a cookie and slowly raised my hand to reach my mouth. By this time, I was already chewing and swallowing without any signs of choking. I was very alert and wanted to be where the action took place. By Christmastime in 1966, I was able to sit up on my own and used my hands to play. My mom felt blessed that my health had improved, since she now felt that I'd be safe in the care of my older sisters or my grandmother.

During my mom's ninth month of pregnancy, three weeks before her due date, she asked her older brother, Maximiliano (nicknamed Chano), to take her to Tepehuanes for a general examination. She had not been feeling well and was concerned about the pregnancy. She left us all in the care of Mama Petra and firmly reminded my sisters not to leave me unattended. My mom had spent the previous months watching me day and night, so she was still apprehensive about leaving me.

My uncle went with her to Tepehuanes and took her to the clinic. During this visit, my mom was examined by a doctor and was told that there appeared to be complications with this pregnancy and that it was necessary for her to have a C-section. Her other eight pregnancies had had no complications and had gone to full term, so this news was concerning. The doctor told her that the C-section would have to be done in Durango because they didn't have the necessary equipment there. My uncle Chano arranged to take her to Durango. The two-hour trip was so stressful that by the time they arrived at the hospital she was in labor. The doctors had to perform an emergency C-section. The delivery lasted hours, and my brother Enrique (Rique) was born. My younger brother was born in February, exactly a year after I contracted polio. My mom was weak but insisted on leaving the hospital the very next day because she was concerned about the rest of us back home.

My mom arrived in La Purísima still weak from the ordeal. She was on bed rest, as was customary for women after giving birth, especially with a C-section. She felt so fatigued and lacked all types of energy. It was a challenge for her to even hold her newborn son to breastfeed him. She just didn't feel right. After a few weeks, she had become feverish and couldn't even manage to stand without feeling like she was going to pass out. She was also having severe pain around her abdomen. My mom wondered if her C-section incision had become infected. Mama Petra convinced my mom to go to Tepehuanes to see what was wrong. Again, my Uncle Chano took my mom into the city.

The doctor examined my mom, and her fever was extremely high. He examined her abdomen, and my mom cringed when he pressed the left side. The doctor told my mom and uncle that he recommended that they go to Durango for an ultrasound and further tests to see what was wrong. Again, my uncle and mom traveled the well-known route to Durango. The doctor immediately ordered tests. He explained, "The C-section does not appear to be infected so I'm ordering other tests to see what could be causing the fever and pain." As my mom went through each exam, she felt sicker by the minute. Once the ordered exams were performed, the doctor came in and shared his diagnosis.

Dr. Madero explained, "During the C-section, the operating doctor unintentionally tied one of your kidneys due to the complicated birth." Apologetically he went on, "As a result, one of your kidneys has stopped working. This kidney failure is what is causing your fever and excruciating pain." Without giving my mom a chance to respond, he said, "The only solution would be to remove the affected kidney since it has stopped working completely."

Dr. Madero was emphatic and said, "I am sorry, but there are more risks if you don't have the surgery, though the surgery can be life threatening." In addition, the doctor spelled out the dangers of such a serious procedure: "The hope is that the right kidney does the work for both kidneys once the left kidney is removed." When the doctor observed my mom's despair, in his attempt to instill hope, he explained, "There have been many cases where other individuals have lived many years with only one kidney, which I hope will be true for you also." My mom, even with her pain and the bad news, kept thinking about her newborn son, me and my recovery, and my other siblings, worrying about our well-being. My uncle kept reminding my mom that she had to get well to be able to care for her children.

My mom didn't want to make the decision about having her kidney removed without my dad's knowing about the situation and without his input. She asked if it could be arranged for her to make a long-distance call to Chicago. The call was arranged, and both my mom and uncle tried to explain the options that were shared with them. My mom was strong but voiced her worries about what would happen with her nine children. My dad listened to what had caused the medical emergency and what had been done to cause the kidney failure. He was adamant about not wanting my mom to have such a serious procedure in the same hospital that had caused the problem. He said, "I don't care about the cost, but I want the best doctors that could do the operation. Please find out who that is. I will be flying to Durango on the first flight I can get."

My uncle asked Dr. Madero for a referral to the best hospital in Mexico that could do the surgery. Dr. Madero fully understood the lack of trust after what had happened. He told my uncle that he would do some research and come back to talk to them the next day. My mom was so weak she didn't have the energy to even voice any questions. In addition, she had been sedated to ease some of the pain. Without realizing, she closed her eyes. All that was in her mind was praying for God's mercy since she didn't want to abandon her family. My uncle sat by her bedside. They were very close, so the possibility of losing his sister really scared him.

The next day, my dad arrived at Durango. Fortunately, he had received his legal residency, so it was much easier for him to travel. When Dr. Madero came to the room, he found my dad sitting next to my mom, though she could barely open her eyes from the pain.

Dr. Madero shared, "Your best option is to go to Juárez, Chihuahua, to a hospital that has done this type of procedure in the past." He continued, "The surgery is expensive and would cost about $25,000 pesos" (about $1,500 U.S. dollars). My dad didn't care about the cost, because all he wanted was the best doctors to help my mom. Dr. Madero reassured my dad and told him, "I will go and arrange everything so that your wife can be transported to Juárez." The trip would take all day since Juárez was about 650 miles from Durango. My dad held my mom's hand as she moaned in pain and couldn't even talk. My dad told my uncle, "Please return to La Purísima and watch over my family. I promise, I will not leave Virginia for a second and will remain by her side."

My mom and dad had never been to Juárez. The city seemed so busy with people coming and going. The hospital was much bigger, though not as big as the ones in Chicago, and this brought more hope to my dad. As Dr. Madero indicated, the hospital was waiting for my mom. They had the surgery scheduled for early the next morning. They gave my mom a room in the intensive care unit. My dad, tired from the long day, sat on a small couch, and held my mom's hand. Each time he was about to doze off, it never failed that a nurse would come to check on my mom. She was on an IV with medication and sedatives. My dad had not slept for over twenty-four hours but knew the next day would be the most difficult.

At 6 AM, a team of doctors came and talked to my dad before taking my mom in for the surgery. They explained, "The surgery will be long because we will carefully remove her entire left kidney." My dad just stared, not wanting to ask the questions that concerned him. Shortly afterward, they came to take my mom, but my dad stopped them so that he could kiss her first. He bent down and gave her a gentle kiss and said in a low voice, "Everything will be OK. God will protect you. I love you." He stood motionless as they carted my mom away.

In the meantime, back in La Purísima, with guidance from Mama Petra, my oldest sister Silveria (Bella) took care of my newborn brother

Rique while my two other sisters watched over me. Mama Petra knew that a nearby neighbor had just had a baby also, so she asked her if she could breastfeed my brother as well. My sister Bella would take Rique three times a day to be fed by the neighbor. The neighbor was also kind enough to share some milk that could be given to my brother with a bottle. My sisters also helped Mama Petra to prepare meals for the whole family; they would always make sure that I ate first before they ate themselves. They had to quickly learn and adjust with my mom's absence. My Uncle Chano told Mama Petra, "I don't know how long Virginia will be in Juárez because they are treating her kidney." To keep Mama Petra from worrying, he didn't share the risks of the surgery or how dangerous it could be.

Back in Juárez, my dad decided to go to a nearby chapel as he waited for my mom's surgery to be over. The chapel was near the hospital, around the corner. The first thing he noticed were the beautiful stained-glass windows around the chapel. The chapel only had about ten rows of pews, and in the center was a large crucifix. He walked in and went to the front row and kneeled. He immediately began to pray, not being aware that he was praying out loud, "Dios, please protect Virginia. All our kids need her. You know that Cuali needs her like no one else, but all our children need their mom. You know I cannot do this alone. Please bless her." He remembered me, and the last time he saw me, when I was still totally paralyzed. Although he knew I had begun to recover some movement, he still had that image of me and knew I needed my mom more than anyone.

He closed his eyes and promised, "I will always be the best husband and dad." His eyes became watery, and a deep sigh escaped. My dad then went silent as he sat in the pew. He suddenly felt a breeze and smelled a soft scent. He looked at the pew where he was sitting and saw a little lavender blossom next to him. He was sure it was not there when he first came in. He looked all around and tried to figure out where this small flower had come from. After looking around and not finding any possible source of the blossom, he picked it up and smelled it. Indeed, it was fresh, for it still had a sweet aroma of lavender. My dad was full of wonderment and felt an overwhelming sense of peace and knew this was God's sign that he had listened to my dad's pleas. I totally believe that indeed this was God's way of sending a message. I am glad my dad took the time to notice the miracle, which sometimes in our hurry we may miss.

After staying at the chapel for a long while, he went back to the hospital's waiting room. He noticed in a corner there was a desk with a little empty glass bottle he assumed had been used for ink. He asked one of the nurses, "May I have this little bottle?" The nurse, confused as to why he would ask when the bottle was obviously trash, replied, "Yes, you may have it." He grabbed it and put the lavender flower in it. He put the small bottle in his pocket and waited patiently, reassured, with faith that the surgery would be a success and that my mom would recover fully. The entire surgery took about seven hours, but to my dad, who waited all alone, it seemed much longer. The doctor finally came and said, "The surgery went well and without complication. However, the next forty-eight hours will be crucial in finding out if the remaining kidney functions in place of two."

What my dad took as God's message in the chapel via the fallen blossom was indeed true. My mom's remaining kidney was functioning perfectly. My mom had a long road to recovery, but the doctor's prognosis was excellent. My dad had felt so angry for the mistake the doctors in Durango made which caused the kidney's failure, but that anger suddenly disappeared. My dad didn't pursue a malpractice suit against the hospital in Durango because of the blossom and the miracle he believes he received after thinking that he was going to lose my mom. It was as if the miracle erased any resentment or anger, so he decided to put this nightmare experience behind him for good.

The first couple of weeks of my mom's recovery were very painful, but even worse was my mom's worry about us in La Purísima. My dad stayed by her side almost entirely. A week after her surgery when her life was no longer in danger, he rented a small room where he stayed at night. My mom received physical therapy for a couple of weeks and then was discharged. She had gotten very weak after the two-month ordeal. She worked hard to regain her strength so that she could return to her family.

My parents returned to La Purísima after six weeks in Juárez. She missed all of us but was most worried about my younger brother and me. They arrived back just a few days before my second birthday. She received all types of hugs and kisses from everyone. My mom commented how we all had grown. She couldn't believe that I was moving my arms so well. My sisters had me show her how I had learned to crawl in a sitting position using my arms. She kissed my baby brother and couldn't believe how big he was after just a couple of months. She told my dad, "We need to baptize him as soon as possible." My dad responded, "I will go arrange it so it can happen tomorrow since I must return to Chicago in the next couple of days."

During the long stay in Juárez, my parents had had a lot of time to plan out what was best for the family. My dad hoped that he could bring us all to Chicago as soon as possible. He convinced my mom to allow my two oldest sisters, Bella and Maria de los Angeles (Angelita), to go back with him so that, between the three of them working, they could save money faster. He told my mom that they would stay with him and that he would find them work in the factory where he currently was employed. Although my mom was hesitant at first, the thought of us all being united was exciting, so she agreed to the plan. When Bella, who was almost seventeen, and Angelita, who was turning fifteen, were informed about the plan, they were excited that they would be traveling to Chicago.

Saying farewell to my dad and two sisters was so difficult for my mom. She prayed that they had made the right decision. She reminded my dad to take care of my sisters and then said, "Girls, if you are not happy for any reason, tell your dad so that you can come back home." My dad had worked on getting permits for them so they could enter the United States, and he was in the process of getting legal residency for the entire family. His goal was to have everyone in Chicago within three or four years. Originally, he had wished he could make it happen in just a couple of years, but with the costs of my mom's surgery, my dad was in debt to his two brothers that worked with him in Chicago and had to pay them back. My mom cried silently each night as she sent blessings to my two sisters who were so far away. She prayed that everyone's sacrifice would be worth it.

CHAPTER 4

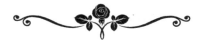

The next four years were long for my mom. She missed my dad and two daughters but knew it was the sacrifice they had to make if we were ever to be reunited. Caring for the rest of us made the time go a bit more quickly, though.

I had learned to get around by crawling, or more like scooting, in a sitting position. My mom couldn't keep up with all my torn pants! She had to sew them in thicker layers by using leftover fabric from the other clothing she made for us. I was so active that she constantly had a needle in her hand. Even without the use of my legs, I had fun playing around, acting like a normal child of my age. The dirt roads of la Purísima, roaming pigs, and rocky terrain didn't stop me. Everyone would treat me as part of the group, helping me when I needed the help. The whole town would just admire how the polio didn't stop me.

It was common for my sister Francisca (Kika), who was twelve years old, to carry me on her back. In fact, Kika often coached me to ask my mom if we could go places because Kika knew that my mom wouldn't say no to me. She also taught me how to act like I was crying when my mom wouldn't give us permission. We sat down under a tree and she said, "Cuali, tell mom that you want to go play lotería. If she says no, rub your eyes and act like you are crying until she says yes." Kika loved to play lotería, the Mexican version of bingo that's played with pictures instead of numbers. Because I enjoyed being around my sister's friends, of course I obliged. No matter where we went, I was given many sweet treats so that I could be entertained. Kika would carry me on her back up and down the whole town and take me to her friends' houses no matter how far they lived. I was too little to understand the games they played but loved being out and about. Kika has wondered if carrying me on her back caused her to stop growing. She is the shortest in the family next to me.

At age five, after seeing how my sister carried me around on her back, my mom thought that maybe she could take me to school too. She knew I was intelligent and didn't want me to miss out on that opportunity. So Kika took the long mile walk with me on her back, sitting down on sidewalks to rest. The walk was long and tiresome. Teresa, nicknamed Tere, would sometimes help too by waiting around until school was over to bring me home. I started kindergarten while Kika was in sixth grade. The two classrooms were on opposite sides of the school. There weren't many classrooms, but the early grades—kindergarten, first, second, and third—were on one side of the building, while grades fourth, fifth, and sixth were on the other. Because la Purísima had no running water, outhouses were used for all grades.

I don't have many memories of my childhood in Mexico, but I do remember my first day of school. My sister left me in my classroom and told the teacher she would be back to take me home. Of course, my sister didn't count on the day being so long and my need to possibly use the bathroom. After a couple of hours, I told my teacher, "Maestra, tengo que orinar (pee)." My teacher knew that I had a cousin in the classroom, so she asked my cousin Cruz to go get my sister Reyna who was in third grade. Joyfully, my cousin Cruz skipped out of the class to go find my sister. With all innocence, Cruz marched into the class and loudly announced, "Cuali quiere cagar (Cuali wants to poop)." My sister wanted to die. She was so embarrassed as the entire classroom started laughing out loud. The teacher tried to settle the class back down as she excused my sister to go help me. Kika's attempt to take me to school only lasted for a week. After the week was up, the family concluded that it was just too difficult.

I wasn't disappointed with the decision to stop; I loved being able to just play. Plus, I was embarrassed to go back because my sister said everyone laughed because I wanted to go poop.

But I didn't feel different. The word disability was never in anyone's vocabulary, much less mine. Everyone looked out for me and never excluded me, accepting me exactly how I was. I loved it and never felt inferior to others. Although I was only five, I was confident and never questioned why I was different.

Everyone in La Purísima was amused by my personality and how my inability to walk didn't deter me from getting to where I needed to go. One day, a man nicknamed Kiko saw how I was playing in the dirt, catching mayates (black beetles) and tying them on a string to make them fly. Kiko saw how dirty I was from all the scooting I had done to get around. Perhaps out of compassion, he built a cart-like device for me to be pulled around in. He took a piece of wood about three feet long and three feet wide and put four wheels on the bottom, then tied on a rope that could be used to pull me. His invention was a hit! Kids loved pulling me around. At first my mom was apprehensive, but when she saw that the invention was sturdy and kept me from getting so dirty, she enjoyed watching me so happy. Over time, the cart's wheels got rusty from all the mud and began making loud noises, so everyone knew when I was coming. Not funny, but some people would say, "Ay viene la pedorra. (Here comes the farter.)" I am glad that nickname didn't stick.

Another memory of my early years was seeing myself on top of my house's roof. I vaguely remember this, and I even thought it was a dream. I didn't remember how I got to the top or what I was doing there, but many years later, my family confirmed that indeed I had been on top of the house, and that it was not a dream. Laughing as they reminisced, they described how my sisters liked playing on the roof with their rag dolls and didn't want to exclude me, so they figured out how to get me to the top. They had used rope to pull me up, wrapping it around my chest. I didn't weigh much so they said it was not too difficult. And then they tied me to my sister so that I wouldn't fall. Of course, when my mom found out, her heart dropped, and she gave my sisters a good spanking.

Likewise, I have a memory of being high up on a hill in front of a huge cross and being able to look down and see the tops of rows of houses. Again, I thought it was a dream, but just as my sisters had figured out how to get me on top of the roof, they also figured how to get me up to "La Cruz" (The Cross). Many years ago, when La Purísima first came to be, a huge Cross made from cement was built on top of the highest point of the town. Since then, La Cruz has come to be an icon of La Purísima, a must-see for any visitor. It was very difficult to get up to La Cruz, more so back then, because there was no established path until very recently. So, it's amazing that I got to the top at all. But this is yet another example of how I lived a very normal childhood.

Because of me, my poor sisters were often victims of reprimands or the "flying huarache (sandal)" several times. Though I don't personally remember it, one time my sister Tere and her friend were knitting and crocheting pillowcases at my paternal uncle's farm, sitting near a wooden trough of water for the animals. My sister Kika arrived with me on her back. She sat me near the trough and started to goof around. It only took a minute of my sisters' distraction for me to fall over, landing right in the trough, and getting completely drenched. My sister Tere quickly pulled me out, but I was soaked through. Tere attempted to dry me off when suddenly my mom arrived. Seeing that I was all wet, she grabbed me from Tere's arms. My mom scolded her and ordered her to take off her skirt so I could be wrapped in it for the walk home. Tere followed, walking quickly, totally embarrassed because all she had on underneath was her slip. Tere remembers that day vividly and believes that my mother punished her without deserving it simply because she was older than Kika.

As I got older, it became obvious that I needed medical care and medical equipment to make my mobility easier. Even though I was now six years old, crawling was still my only way to move from one place to another. And because of all the crawling, my legs fused in one position, and my joints were very stiff. I also had callused hands from always scrambling around in the dirt. After my slightly disastrous attempt to go to school, my mom urged my dad to reunite the family as soon as possible. My dad kept asking my mom to have patience. He and my two sisters were working hard and saving every penny. My sisters never went out; their checks were always given entirely to my dad. Not to mention, my dad was still waiting on immigration to approve the application for legal residency for all of us so that he could bring us to Chicago. But he had already rented a small house in the Humboldt Park neighborhood in Chicago where mostly Latinos lived. Both of my parents were fully aware of the urgency of bringing me to the United States. They knew that this would be my only hope for a future.

My dad eventually received the good news that we were to present ourselves to the United States immigration office to receive our legal residency. My dad had been concerned about my polio being an obstacle for me to receive legal residency, so he made sure to discuss it with his lawyer. She reassured him that because it was no longer contagious and because my mental capacity had not been affected, there should be no issue. My dad was so relieved to know that there would be no problem, especially because I was one of the main reasons why we were moving to a different country.

My dad and sisters made the plans for our move to Chicago. My dad had a sister, Tia Maria de Jesus, whom we call Tia Chuy, who helped with all the preparations by figuring out the necessary sleeping arrangements for a family of eleven. She lived nearby and had friends who donated blankets, pillows, and even a couple of mattresses. My dad and sisters shopped for winter clothing since it was December and we would all need warm clothes once we arrived in Chicago. They made sure to have all the necessary permits, and then purchased two round-trip tickets for my sisters and eight one-way tickets to Chicago for the rest of us. My dad stayed in Chicago to ensure everything was ready for our arrival. They were so excited that it was hard for them to work and even harder to sleep.

When my mom was notified by telegram that my sisters would be arriving and that we would all be going to Chicago, she began her own preparations. She gave all her chickens to Mama Petra who was sadly staying behind. She made sure to ask my uncle Chano to keep an eye on the house, which she was leaving locked up. She gave some of our old clothes to other families. Every night, as she got us in bed, she would tell us how she imagined Chicago to be and warned us about how cold it was. Of course, she just shared what she imagined since she had never left Mexico in her life. What I remember most vividly was her explanation of our skin color. She said, "In Chicago, people are light skinned because the sun is far. Here we are dark skinned because the sun burns us." We were all eager to know what Chicago was really like.

Time went by quickly with all she had to do, and before she knew it, my sisters were in La Purísima to come and get us. My mom was so happy to see my sisters and kept commenting on how much they had changed. They unpacked all the coats and scarfs and tried them on, laughing at how we looked. One of my sisters told us, "All of us are getting into a HUGE airplane that will take us to Chicago." My other sister chimed in, excitely saying, "When the plane takes off it goes really fast and then it lifts the front wheels until the plane is up in the sky. Your stomach may feel weird and your ears will pop." We just couldn't believe that we would be up in the sky. As we talked during our last day in La Purísima, my mom outlined all that we would have to do when we got to Chicago. "Lo primero es la escuela (The first thing is school)," she said. Then she said, "Your dad has found a good hospital for Cuali, and his insurance can help pay for the costs." That comment reminded my mom to tell me, "Don't forget not to crawl around. I will carry you." We all nodded in agreement and my mom said, "You all have to behave and listen to me. In the airport, there are a lot of people."

My mom carried me all the way until I arrived in Chicago on December 15, 1971. Some people who saw my mom carrying me jokingly said, "Young lady, aren't you too big to be carried." Luckily,

I didn't understand them or else I may have opened my mouth and said something I shouldn't have. My mom just smiled and didn't respond because she didn't understand either. The entire trip was mesmerizing. I wish I could remember the flight, but I don't. What I do remember is seeing snow for the first time. I couldn't believe how pretty it looked, but immediately wondered how I would crawl on it. I couldn't imagine how snow would feel.

We loved our new home! Each of us were amazed with different aspects of the house. My brothers loved the bathroom. They must have flushed the toilet a dozen times. On the other hand, I was busy trying to figure out how my mom was able to talk on the phone. I was sure someone was hiding in the closet. I crawled to open the nearby closet door to ensure that the person she was talking to was not in there. We felt like we had gone from rags to riches. Our refrigerator was amazing. It had two doors and it was full of food. We couldn't believe that we could keep food in the fridge for a long time.

The TV was unbelievable. We had never watched television before. We would try to mimic speaking in English like the actors on screen. My brother would say "gibberish, gibberish." And my sister would respond, "gibberish, gibberish." As we explored the different channels, some shows were immediate hits. We all fell in love with The Three Stooges, perhaps because we didn't need to know English to know what was happening, and we found it funny. I do remember struggling to figure out how the TV worked. We only had a black and white set, and the dial was used to change the channel. However, we didn't realize that the shows fell on a certain schedule and on a certain channel. Every morning, we would turn the dial slowly until we found the Stooges. Sometimes it would take multiple times around the dial until we saw the Stooges and not a commercial. We would also take turns in holding the V-shaped antenna a certain way to get the best picture, until we discovered that aluminum foil could hold the antenna in place. Because it was just a few days until the holidays, we didn't have to worry about school yet. We were enjoying our new home, waking up each morning to the Stooges and our box of "con-fleis" (corn flakes, the word my mom used for all cereal).

Our sleeping arrangements were unconventional, since it was not easy to fit eleven people into a small two-bedroom house. We moved into the second floor of a three-floor building. We had to be careful how much noise we made because another family lived below us. After all the warnings from our parents, I think the mice made more noise than we did.

My dad had already discovered the problem with mice, so he had bought mouse traps to capture them. I remember one night, when we were all in bed with the lights out, the mice were more active than ever. Some of us were already falling asleep when a trap caught a mouse, making a loud SNAP. My oldest brother, Mon, couldn't resist and yelled, "Uno! (One!)" Soon after, another mouse was caught and again made a loud SNAP. I am not sure which sister yelled out "Dos! (Two!)" but I believe we got to siete (seven) before my dad quieted us down. In the morning, we all wanted to see the victims, but my parents had already gathered the mice and took them out to the trash in our alley.

We celebrated our first Christmas a short ten days after arriving in Chicago, and we have continued with this yearly tradition since then. My parents always felt that Christmas was the most important holiday to be together as a family. My sisters had bought a Christmas tree when they lived with my dad before we were all reunited. It was a bright silver tinsel tree that was about four feet high. I had never seen a more beautiful tree. I loved how the lights reflected on the tinsel to form a rainbow array of colors. Most of us still believed in El niñito Dios (infant Jesus) who brought us sweets and presents if we were good. The image of Santa Claus was new to us and it wasn't until we were in school that we joined the Santa Claus fan club. That Christmas was the most special one I had ever had. It was the first time we were all together. There was more food than ever, and we had presents that were more than an old mended sock filled with candy.

I vaguely remember that I wore a bright red and gold shirt and had a huge smile the entire time. Oh, how I loved to be with my family.

We first lived on a street named St. Louis, and then a year later moved to a slightly bigger house on Kimball, just a couple of streets down. Both of our homes were close to an elementary public school. We were excited because my mom was going to register us for school now that the holidays were over. My aunt Chuy's bilingual friend Matilde agreed to go with my mom to help get us enrolled in school. Because the nine of us ranged in ages from four to twenty, not everyone registered at the elementary school. My mom wanted to register me (aged six), Lalo (aged eight), Reyna (aged ten), Mon (aged eleven), and Kika (aged fourteen). My three oldest sisters were not going to go to school because they were going to work to help support the family.

Mom dressed us all nicely and walked down the street to Stowe Elementary school, a Chicago public school. My mom carried me while she held my baby brother's hand; he was still too young to enter school. The principal registered us in the various grades based on our ages. Of course, we didn't understand anything he was saying except when he mentioned our names. I sat there with my eyes wide open, trying to catch what was being said. I couldn't figure out why my full name "Pascuala" kept being mentioned. It was strange to even hear it because no one ever called me Pascuala. People in my family and in La Purísima always called me Pascualita or Cuali. I looked at my mom, the principal, and Matilde, to see if they would give me a clue about what was going on.

Matilde then explained, "Pascualita cannot go to this school because she has a disability and can't walk." I started to wonder if, yet again, I wouldn't be able to go to school. I wasn't disappointed at the thought, yet I couldn't figure out why they weren't letting me go to their school. I figured that since the school was so close, being carried on my sister's back wouldn't be a problem like it had been in La Purísima. Matilde continued, "She has to go to a special school for kids who have different disabilities." I don't think I had ever heard the word "disability" before. For the first time ever, I felt singled out because I couldn't walk, and now there was a word for it, not just polio. In that split second, it dawned on me that I was different from my brothers and sisters, and that because I couldn't walk, I had to go to another school. I interrupted Matilde and asked, "Por que?" She answered my question but looked at my mom as she responded, "Because she cannot walk, she will be picked up by bus and go to a special school named Spalding that is about ten miles away." I didn't know how I felt, but I knew it didn't feel right. When we got home, Matilde made a phone call. When she hung up, she told us she had arranged for us to go to Spalding School the next day.

CHAPTER 5

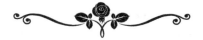

My stomach began to hurt after the phone call to Spalding even though I hadn't eaten too much. Deep down I was feeling upset but couldn't verbalize why. My other siblings were set to go to school, but I wasn't, and I thought that was unfair. My mom wondered if I was feeling anxiety over having to go to school by myself; I had never been apart from at least one person in my family, and things were so different from La Purísima. I asked my mom, "Why can't I go to the school that is close to us?" She didn't give much of a response and just said, "Because you need a special school." That night, it was hard to sleep since I worried about all the new experiences, and I felt so lost not knowing what was going on.

We arrived at Spalding Elementary/High School, the main school attended by individuals with disabilities in Chicago. Immediately, I noticed huge wooden wheelchairs at the entrances and in several corners. My dad had told me I would get a wheelchair in Chicago so I wouldn't have to be carried, but I never imagined them to be so big! They looked scary, not like something that would help me. I also noticed women outside each hallway that looked like nurses, all dressed in white. I almost wanted to ask if this was a hospital instead of a school, but I figured I would find out soon enough, so I remained quiet. I saw some students in the hallway, but they all looked so strange. Some were in helmets, some had walking sticks that reminded me of an old man that lived close to us in La Purísima.

This also was the first time I remembered seeing people who looked different than the people I had seen in La Purísima. I saw students who were light skinned and with different hair color. I also saw black people for the first time in my life. I am sure there were black people in the airport, but the entire trip was a blur to me because of my excitement. In La Purísima I knew a friend that looked much lighter than I did, but not with blonde hair like one of the kids I saw waiting for the elevator as we walked to the principal's office. I also saw kids around my age who walked with metal bars on their legs. In the elevator, when it briefly stopped, I saw a girl in a wheelchair and was relieved that it was a much smaller and prettier chair than the one I saw by the door when we came in.

Some students were being pushed in their chairs, while others were walking with the assistance of someone behind them holding a belt wrapped around them. I later found out that the women dressed in white were not nurses but attendants who were there to help students at mealtime or when going to the bathroom. The school also had physical therapists like the one helping the student walk with a belt around her waist. It felt very scary to me, as if I was in a foreign world. I doubted that I would be able to adjust to this school. However, Matilde helped my mom register me even when I kept hoping they would say I couldn't attend for some reason or another, like my two previous schools had. All I kept saying in my mind was *I want to go home*.

I was so happy to leave the school that day. It was as if I could breathe again. I felt I didn't belong there and hoped both my mom and Matilde would agree. Sadly, based on their conversation, I knew they were not feeling the same way I did, and they wanted me to go back to that awful place. Matilde told my mom that I had to go to the children's hospital to get a wheelchair for school. They talked as if I couldn't hear or understand, but every comment made me more nervous than the previous. On the one hand, I was glad to find out that I wouldn't have to use those ugly wooden wheelchairs and that

I couldn't start school yet. Yet, I was disappointed that they kept talking about their plan for me to attend Spalding.

Matilde suggested we go to Children's Memorial Hospital immediately since we were not too far from it. My mom thought it was a good idea to get as much done as possible, since she hated leaving my younger brother with my Aunt Chuy for too long. Matilde was sure that we would be seen without an appointment if we went to the emergency room. I didn't think things could get any worse, but I was wrong. I was in complete culture shock, not just because of the new language and different races, but also because I was now having to deal with being disabled, being treated as if there were something wrong with me. I started to imagine the worst. I thought to myself, *Am I going to die, and they don't know how to tell me?* It felt odd to think that I had to go to the hospital when I didn't feel sick, beyond having an upset stomach from nervousness. It was as if, suddenly, I wasn't good enough anymore and the goal was to fix me. I had never thought of myself as someone who needed to be fixed.

On the way there, close to the hospital, I looked out the window and saw these beautiful snow-covered lawns. I didn't see many people around since it was January and very cold. I wondered what that place was. A few blocks later we got to Children's Memorial Hospital. It was enormous. Matilde asked a man if I could use a wheelchair; my mom must have been exhausted after carrying me all day. But this wheelchair was not like the wooden one I saw at the school. It was much smaller, and not made of wood. The chair was shiny, and I was able to reach the big wheels, which I was certain I couldn't do on the wooden wheelchairs.

We went inside and Matilde signed us in to see a doctor. She also asked the young woman at the desk who she could talk to about getting financial help to pay for the hospital, because we were not sure if my dad's insurance would cover me. I didn't wait too long before they called me into one of the rooms. My mom lifted me up out of the wheelchair and put me on the examining table. The doctor that came in was tall and had grayish hair but seemed nice because he smiled at me and wanted to shake my hand. He laid me down on the table and examined each of my bones. I was so nervous, and his hands were cold. I wondered what he was looking for. He kept asking me to do things that I didn't understand until Matilde told me what to do. He asked, "Do you feel this?" Matilde translated and I would say "yes" no matter where he touched. He tried to straighten my right leg from the bent position, but he couldn't. My mom told Matilde, "She can't straighten her right leg because of how she scooted around on the ground." Matilde translated as I listened intently, trying to understand anything she was saying.

The doctor stood by the door and said, "We need some X-rays, and I want her to come back in two weeks". Right before stepping out, the doctor said, "One of the priorities is going to be to straighten her right leg, but we can talk about that at our next visit." Matilde reminded the doctor that I needed a wheelchair ordered and asked if he could put a rush on it because I needed it to go to school. Matilde knew that I would qualify for support from agencies such as March of Dimes and Easter Seals because I had a disability. She told my mom that she would apply for us. After we qualified, my dad continued to contribute donations to those two wonderful agencies for many years because of the support they provided. Matilde scheduled the appointment and gave the copies of the appointments for radiology and the doctor to my mom.

While Matilde drove us home, she discussed everything that was decided and other plans she had to help us. Biting my lip, I asked, "When will I go to school?" Matilde said, "As soon as you get your wheelchair." I relaxed knowing that at least for a few days, I would be safe at home with my mom. I was not looking forward to going to school where everyone acted and looked so different. I was also not in favor of going to the hospital again in two weeks. I was still puzzled, not being able to quite comprehend how they would take pictures of my bones like Matilde explained to my mom before she left our house.

My mom may not have been going to the stream to fetch water like she used to, but she was certainly busy. Just grocery shopping was such a different experience. In the past, she would mostly buy what was needed for the day, except for the sacks of beans and rice. However, now that we had a refrigerator, she had to think about everything that she needed for the whole week. She was also not confident about being able to communicate, but she soon found out that there was always someone that could speak both Spanish and English who would gladly help. Not every grocery store sold the Mexican products she needed, but luckily there was a market that wasn't too far that did. I loved going with her, but I did get a lot of stares from people who didn't know the reason why I was being carried or put into carts.

My mom also had to learn how to use the appliances in our home. She found the washing machine to be especially difficult at first, though she was so grateful for not having to wash by hand. She would comment, "These clothes don't come out as clean as when I washed them by hand." My older siblings had started their routine in school and every afternoon they would share the words they learned in English. I was sad that I couldn't go to school with them.

My sister Kika was in eighth grade and was going to graduate that coming June. The family needed more income, though, so it was decided that she would go to work instead of going to high school. (She did later finish her GED.) She was a quick learner and picked up English at work, always moving up in responsibilities and making more money. My dad didn't know how to drive, and though he had learned how to use the Chicago Transit Authority (CTA) bus system, he found a coworker that drove them to work if my dad gave him money for gas. My dad never did learn how to drive, especially not after his children became drivers.

My mom had so many appointments to get me the help I needed. She applied for financial support for my medical care, which I was approved for immediately, thanks to a combination of my disability, because we were such a huge family, and because my dad didn't earn much income. She also took me to an appointment to be measured for a wheelchair, which was delivered a week later. Then, she took me back to the hospital to see the doctor again and to get the X-rays he had ordered.

Having X-rays was such a weird experience. The table was so cold that I shivered when I had to lay on it. The lady also asked me to get into different positions while she placed big frames under me and moved a huge machine over parts of my legs. When she noticed I didn't know what she was saying, she moved me how she wanted. If I couldn't get into the position she wanted me to be, she used pillows, tape, and heavy weights to hold me there. I really didn't need to know English because the lady would just move me the way she wanted, mumbling words I didn't understand. The only words that she said in Spanish, with her American accent, were "no respira (no breathing)" and "respira (breathe)".

After taking the X-rays, we went to meet with the doctor. I was already tired, hungry, and wanted to go home. My mom pulled out a homemade tortilla de harina (flour tortilla) from her purse and said, "Ya casi." I knew I had to be patient. The doctor called us in and immediately began to say, "I looked at the X-rays and I think it is important to straighten her right knee so we can look to see if she could walk with braces." Matilde translated and my mom was clearly excited about me possibly walking. I would have been excited, but I was worried about what they had to do. He said, "I want to schedule a surgery to straighten her leg, but the process will be long and difficult." Matilde was interpreting for my mom, giving her the details of the surgery. My ears were wide open as my heart started to beat faster and faster. I didn't like the plan because my mom was told that I would have to be in the hospital for a long time. My mom knew I was getting anxious, so she just looked at me as if to say *Be strong and don't cry*. When I looked back at my mom, though, it was obvious that she was trying to be strong, too. She just nodded to the explanation Matilde was giving her. If she had any questions, she didn't dare to ask them.

The surgery was scheduled for just a little over a month after we first arrived in Chicago, for the first week in February. My mom was worried about the delay in my starting school but was told that I would get some schooling in the hospital during my recovery and then go to Spalding afterward. Even though I was already anxious, it had not hit me that I would be all alone in the hospital. I had no idea what was coming. When Matilde and my Aunt Chuy took us to the hospital, it was very grey and snowy. The weather matched my mood. Again, I wasn't sure why it was so important for me to have my leg straightened. For as long as I could remember, my leg had been this way and it didn't bother me. Still, I had to trust my mom and just be strong.

I am not exactly sure how long the surgery lasted, but it seemed to be quick. The last thing I remembered was my mom hugging me as I was taken to the operating room. When I woke up, I noticed that my leg was straight, and it looked and felt strange. The leg was all bandaged but not in a cast. I was very sleepy still and wasn't nervous or in any pain. I was looking for my mom and began to feel scared as the nurses were talking to me as if I understood everything. Two men took me through a long hallway; I remember the bright lights on the ceiling. I started to cry quietly, not knowing where I was being taken.

When we arrived, I was so relieved to see my mom but kept crying anyway. They had taken me to what would be my home for the next thirty-one days. However, it was nothing like my real home where I felt safe and loved. This room was cold, sad, painful, and I hated it. The two men carefully slid me onto another bed in the room. They said something which neither my mom nor I understood. My mom noticed my puzzled face and said, "Your Aunt Chuy and Matilde went downstairs to eat when they told us you were out of the surgery." When the two men left, she asked, "Come te sientes?" All I could do was cry. She just brushed my hair back with her hand and gently told me, "Mija, vas a poder caminar. Es por tu bien." Even if I was going to be able to walk and it was for my own good, I didn't like it. We were happy that my aunt and Matilde came back when the nurse returned to the room. My mom had noticed that even my left foot was bandaged, and it was something she didn't expect. What startled her most was seeing a long stainless-steel nail going through each of my heels. She didn't say anything because I had not noticed this, and she didn't want to alarm me.

The bed had a huge bar on the top with a triangle dangling down. I had noticed it and wondered what it was for, but I was too scared to even ask. The nurse then started talking as she moved and adjusted the bar on top of the bed and pulled what seemed like elastic ropes. She said, "The triangle is to help her sit up when she feels better." She then said, "Sorry, this is going to hurt." She then tied the ropes to each of the nails that pierced my heels. She told Matilde, "This treatment is called traction, and each day, we will add more weight so that her legs can be stretched and straightened." As she tied the ropes, I started crying, and by this time, I didn't care to be strong anymore. I screamed for her to stop and yelled, "No me gusta. Ama dígales que no." My mom was suffering as she gulped, telling me to calm down. I pleaded, "Me duele!" It was painful! I had never felt this type of pain, not even the time I had fallen off the cart that Kiko made for me.

In the evening, my dad and three sisters came after work. They brought me a stuffed animal and a balloon, but I didn't even care. I was still very upset. Matilde and my aunt had left by then, so my mom tried to explain what they were doing to straighten my legs. My dad asked, "Why the left leg too?" My mom didn't know herself but said, "Maybe that leg was also stiff?" They tried to take my mind off my legs and pain, but I couldn't forget.

After a couple of hours, my dad said in a quiet voice, "We should go home because we might not find a taxi later." My eyes opened wide. What? Were they all going to leave me? I lost it. I started to scream from the top of my lungs. "No me dejen! (Don't leave me!)" I clung to my mom's coat as my dad tried to pull her away. They all left crying. I cried until I couldn't anymore. My parents and sisters cried as much as I did that night. They prayed that this was what was best for me.

For thirty-one days, the agony continued. I became very angry and even started to use cuss words I had never used. I screamed, begging for them to let me die. I told every doctor or nurse that I hated them. Perhaps as a manipulative tactic, I also told my family that I hated them for leaving me. I know that it became harder and harder for my mom to come. She had even asked if she could stay overnight, but my dad reminded her that the rest of the kids, especially Rique, needed her to be home with them. I wasn't eating the hospital food. My mom got permission to bring me food from home. She hoped it would make me feel better, but it didn't.

During the days, people came and went. One of them must have been a teacher because she had me copy out different letters. I already knew how to write some letters because my older brothers and sisters had taught me, and I was happy to see that the letters were the same in both English and Spanish. I learned how to spell my full name, even though everyone in my family still just called me Cuali. On the 30th day, they took me to another room and again put me to sleep. I didn't know that they were taking out the nails running through my heels. They bandaged my left foot and casted my right leg from my toes to the top of my thigh. I didn't care about the cast or bandage; all I cared about was that I would be going home the next day!

We were discharged, and my dad asked my Uncle Jesus, my Aunt Chuy's husband, whom we also called Chuy, to pick us up. My dad carefully lifted and stretched me out in the back seat of the car. My mom and aunt sat in the front seat with my uncle while my dad squeezed into a small corner in the back. We were welcomed home by my family with drawings, balloons, and cookies. They all cheered for me and told me how cool my cast was. They were also excited to show me my new wheelchair. They said, "look, it can go fast." I was not excited. I was tired and just wanted to watch TV.

The hospital arranged for a teacher to come to our house for homeschooling. It was a different teacher than the one in the hospital. I had begun to learn a few English words but still couldn't even form a sentence. Luckily the teacher was bilingual so my mom could talk to her directly. She told my mom, "I am going to come three times a week for two hours." My mom asked, "For how long?" She replied, "The order is for six weeks."

Throughout the six weeks we worked on many things. We did subjects like spelling, math, and even drawing. I liked the teacher and what I was learning. It was also a good distraction because being in bed all day was starting to get boring. Sometimes, I would be carried to the living room, but I preferred being in bed. I couldn't wait until I could go outside now that the weather was getting better. But it seemed like the only place I would ever go was to the hospital for my appointments.

Because I couldn't yet get up, I had to use a bedpan to go to the bathroom. One morning I yelled out to my mom, and when she came in, I said, "I want to use the bathroom." She brought the bedpan and I lifted myself and made room for her to slide it under me. As I started to urinate, someone was at the door. We had forgotten that the teacher had changed her schedule, so we were not expecting her. When I heard the teacher's voice, I quickly grabbed the sheet and covered myself. Both my mom and I were too embarrassed to let the teacher know that I needed a minute to get the bedpan out. Instead, I had my entire school lesson with that thing under me. I don't think I'd ever been so focused and compliant before. I thought that the more I focused, the shorter my lesson would be. I will never forget this experience; how could I? I was on the bed pan for two *long* hours. It was torture. My homeschool teacher never found out that I had been using the bathroom during the entire lesson.

After six weeks, the day finally came for them to take my cast off. I was so excited. I was tired of my sponge baths and the itchiness I felt at night. They used a special saw, and I was scared they might also cut through my skin. It made a loud noise as if they were digging on concrete. The more they drilled, the hotter my leg got. If I wasn't so scared, I would have giggled because it tickled a little bit. They sawed two lines, one on each side, from top to bottom. They then used a tool to push the top and bottom pieces of the cast. It felt weird for them to pull the cast off, yet I felt relieved. I was crying, more because of fear, and less because of pain—that is, until they slowly bent my leg. Then, I was crying in pain. After two months of being straight, now my leg had gotten used to it and didn't want to bend. The doctor told my mom, "You will need to do these exercises at home. Before bed, bend her leg like this at least ten times. She will also need therapy."

At home, I guarded my leg as a precious treasure. I was afraid of it being hurt or bent. I knew that I could no longer crawl like I used to because my leg now wanted to be straight. I was not used to my wheelchair either, so I felt trapped. My mom would want to do the movements the doctor told her to do with my leg, but I begged her not to. Each time she would say, "It's for your own good."

She never listened to my begging. One day, while she was doing the exercises, she said, "Mija, you start school on Monday. A bus will pick you up at 7:30 in the morning." Before I could object, she continued saying, "They are doing therapy there, so the more you bend the leg, the less it will hurt." I knew there was no way I could change her mind, so I dreaded Monday for three whole days.

CHAPTER 6

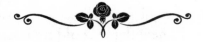

T he first day of school was short! The bus came right on time at 7:30 AM sharp. My mom had to carefully bring me down in my wheelchair from the second floor. I was still light enough for her to do that, but I knew she would struggle as I got bigger. The bus was yellow and much smaller than I expected. A platform came out and the bus driver put me on it. After putting on my wheelchair brakes, I got lifted into the bus, where an attendant was waiting for me. She moved my chair into position and then strapped me in. I was so anxious and in despair that I yelled out for my mom, "Ama, no quiero ir." I begged my mom to let me stay home. I pleaded again, "Por favor, no quiero ir a la escuela. (Please, I don't want to go to school.)" My mom pretended to not hear me and started going up the stairs.

The door closed, and I started to feel nauseous. We stopped to pick up three other kids from their homes, but I felt horrible throughout the whole trip. I was going to tell the lady that I felt like throwing up but didn't know how to do it. Before I knew it, I threw up and it went all over my clothes. We were almost at the school and I saw the attendant say something to the driver. I was hoping she had said to take me back home, but when the bus didn't turn around, I realized they were still headed to the school. The other students looked disgusted and kept staring at me. When we got to the school, I was taken to the nurse. The nurse asked for a Spanish speaker to call my mom to tell her that I had gotten sick and that they were taking me back home. I was relieved.

As soon as I got home, I felt better. I even felt hungry because I had not eaten breakfast in the morning as a protest against having to go to school. I watched TV with my brother until my other siblings got home. My mom was puzzled, and though she wondered what she should do, still she said, "Mañana si vas." I would have to go to school the next day. She added, "If you eat breakfast, you will not get sick." I wasn't thrilled that I would have to face the bus and go to school again the next day.

For days, I kept getting sick. After bringing me home several times, my mom told the nurse to leave me in school because I had not shown any signs of being sick at home. They told her that they couldn't keep me because I had soiled my clothes. So back home I went. And again, I was perfectly fine when I got home. My mom was now angry at me, thinking that I was faking it just to come home. Either that or my nerves were causing me to get sick. Either way, she felt she had to find a solution. She decided to pack an extra set of clothes in my backpack without telling me. The next day, I threw up again and when she was called, she told them to please change me and leave me at school. I finally had my first full day of school.

I wish I could say that I liked my first day of school, but I hated it. I didn't understand anything that was going on and especially hated lunchtime. I wasn't used to all this strange looking food—I didn't see beans, rice, tacos, or any of the food that I was used to. I thought everything looked strange and the smell was too strong. I didn't want to eat at all. During lunch, the attendants would walk around to help those that couldn't eat on their own. One attendant thought I couldn't feed myself when she saw my tray completely untouched. I didn't know how to tell her that my tray was full because I didn't like the food. She picked me up and sat me on her lap and tried to spoon-feed me. I shut my mouth tight and made gagging noises as she put the spoon by my lips. She took this as a challenge and tried to force-feed me. It was awful. She was so angry at me when I won the battle and didn't open my mouth even a little. She picked me up and sat me back on my chair as she left all frustrated.

I didn't enjoy any part of my school day, but lunchtime was the worst. First, I sat with other kids who I didn't know and who didn't speak Spanish. One Latino kid, Elias, started to sit by me. I hoped he spoke Spanish, but he didn't. Instead, he started to bother and take advantage of me, knowing that I couldn't tattle on him because I didn't speak English. He pulled one of my braids, then the other, looking away, pretending it wasn't him. I said, "Ouch, no me hales! (Don't pull!)" He did this every chance he had. I tried to mime what he was doing to snitch on him, but the attendant didn't understand and thought I was just playing with my hair.

As the weeks passed by, the issues in the cafeteria continued. I think that because of me, they started a lunch policy. They decided that every student had to eat their lunch before they could go out for recess. The weather was getting warmer and it was almost my birthday month. I was getting tired of not going out to recess and just sitting there staring at my food. Some attendants felt sorry for me, and secretly threw some of the food in the trash so that I could go to recess. They knew I wouldn't eat it, no matter what it was. But sometimes they couldn't help me because the lunch monitors were nearby.

One day, I really wanted to go to recess, and had a plan! I sat and looked at my food, and thought to myself, if I drop the full tray, I will not have to eat the food. So, I took a quick look around, and when I didn't see anyone, I discreetly pushed the tray off the table. It crashed down loudly, and Ms. Murphy, the meanest lunch monitor, yelled out, "No, no, no!" I was thinking, *Oh no, she saw me*.

Ms. Murphy then grabbed my wheelchair and started pushing me. I didn't know where she was taking me. She wheeled me inside the girls' bathroom, grabbed a bunch of paper towels, and put them on my lap. I wondered why. My heart was pounding. I didn't have a clue what she was going to do. She then pushed me back to the cafeteria, right next to the table where the food tray was still on the floor. No one had dared to clean it up. Ms. Murphy then picked me up out of my wheelchair, abruptly sat me on the floor, and gave me the paper towels so that I could clean the mess. I felt so humiliated. Everyone appeared to be looking at me. From the corner of my eye, I saw the attendant who had helped me throw away some food the previous day. She almost looked like she was crying. I thought, *at any moment, she is going to defend me*. Unfortunately, she didn't. I just kept cleaning the floor. I was crying, but deep down, I was happy that at least my plan worked, and I didn't have to eat the food.

In the evening, I told my mom about the cafeteria experience. First, she said, "La comida no se desperdicia," reminding me that food should not be wasted. Next, she asked me, "Why don't you eat?" I replied, "I don't like the food. It smells and I don't know what it is." She then asked, "Would you eat if you brought food from home?" I quickly responded, "Claro que si." I don't know how she did it, but from then on, everyone got cafeteria food while I got my mom's home-cooked meals. Even the attendants were eager to see what I was having for lunch and wanted a taste of my delicious Mexican food!

My only relief from school and hospitals was evenings and weekends with my family. After applying for immigration, Mama Petra was granted legal residence and she came to live with us. She was fun, carefree, and entertaining. She was a smoker, and when my mom was not watching, she would offer us a puff. Of course, we knew she was kidding. Or at least we thought she was. Having her live with us gave my mom a bit more flexibility in taking me to doctors' appointments. Unfortunately, I never met either of my grandfathers, and my paternal grandmother Tina had died shortly after we moved to Chicago. She had always treated me special and dreamed of my being able to walk. She even admitted that I was her most adored grandchild.

Thankfully, Spalding was not a residential school, or else it wouldn't only feel like a prison; it really would be a prison. At least when I was at home, I could forget about all my troubles and feel normal again. When I arrived home from school, my mom would have two fried eggs ready for me, and she would ask one of my siblings to go get me French fries from a hotdog place on the corner. I loved eating my over-medium eggs with fries. Even as an adult, that was the food of choice my mom would offer me. How I wish I could have those two over-medium eggs and fries again. I think her secret was frying them with lard.

Sometimes my mom would get creative as she was trying to assimilate. She always looked for the Tombstone pizza sales. She would change it up from my usual two eggs with fries and have some Tombstone pizza nice and warm waiting for me. Tombstone pizza would become one of the daily breads in our family. She raised us, her grandchildren, and the neighborhood kids on pizza. Of course, she was the only one that could cook it to a perfect crisp in her busted toaster oven. Even after the toaster oven lost a hinge, she used a wooden spoon to hold the door shut. It must have been her secret because no one else could cook the pizza just like her.

I was close to everyone in my family, but especially my little brother, Rique. I thought he was the most adorable little boy. He was so smart. He knew every single song on every record my sisters had. He still didn't know how to read, but he visually recognized which song was on which record. I loved hanging out with him and would imitate how he couldn't roll his *r*'s but would pronounce them as *l*'s instead. We hung out every Sunday after church. My dad would give each of us a dollar, so we would pool our money and get a bag of O-Ke-Doke popcorn and a bottle of RC Cola. We sat outside when the weather was nice and ate our delicious purchases. Our fingers turned yellow and wrinkly from licking them after each mouthful of popcorn.

I remember one Sunday I ruined the popcorn routine. My dad, as usual, had given us a dollar each. However, he gave me a dollar in coins, and I wanted the dollar bill that he gave Rique. I got mad, and though he explained over and over that we both got the same, in a temper tantrum, I flung the coins to the floor in my brother's direction. My dad was appalled and visibly angry. He picked up the coins, and said, "Now you get nothing. You will not get any more coins or dollar bills until you say sorry to me and your brother." By the following Sunday I had my dollar back and never complained about coins again, even when there were pennies.

I also loved my sisters a lot. My two older sisters were already dating. Sometimes they would ask to go out to a movie or out to eat with their boyfriends, but my parents wouldn't let them go unless they took me and my brother. When we went to the movies, they would convince us to sit in the front while they sat in the back. My sisters would beg to go to dances and would often bribe my parents by cleaning the house and taking me to the park if it wasn't too cold. I was good at keeping secrets if I was rewarded with candy or other goodies. I never told my parents that sometimes the boyfriends would meet them at the park. Not too long after coming to the United States, my oldest sisters got married.

Even after my two sisters got married, they continued to help the family any way they could. Tere was the first one to learn how to drive so she drove us where we needed to go when she was not working. My mom was always the one to take me to doctor appointments because my dad had to work at the factory to make money to pay the rent and other living expenses. My dad started feeling very stressed and was always worried about how he would pay all the bills. I believe this is what led him to increase his drinking. During the weekends, he would drink Hamm's beer until he became an alcoholic. Though he drank more than he should, he always drank at home and never missed work. It was still very hard for my mom to see him drink so heavily. Once Mondays came around, my dad had an enormous regret and would ask my mom for forgiveness. Yet, when Friday came again, he would start the same cycle.

When my dad drank too much, he would become very sentimental. He would love for me to sit with him to talk. He would tell me stories about how much he missed us when he was in the United States without us. He would say, "I want you all to go to school because I never went even one day." Then, he would show off and tell me how he taught himself math and how to read. He said he had read the Bible from front to back several times. He also taught me how the streets in Chicago run. He said, "If you know where Lake Michigan is, you will never get lost." I was so impressed with everything he knew. I didn't know that someday what he taught me would become very handy. Because of him, I was able to learn the whole city and become a virtual Chicago atlas.

My dad never stopped expressing how much we all meant to him, especially my mom. He would get teary and say, "Soy un hombre muy rico." He felt he was the richest man ever because he had my mom and us. He would often tell me about all he hoped for each of us. He would say, "I want you to walk someday and become very successful and make good money because you know Spanish and English." He had a very simplistic way to stress what he wanted for me in my life. He said, "If you know English, have a dollar in your pocket, and have a family that loves you, nothing will stop you from being successful." He said that was his greatest dream. This motivated me and inspired me to work hard to learn English and I knew that an education would be my only way to make his dream come true.

My mom, on the other hand, was not as verbally expressive. She showed that she loved me with actions and not words. She couldn't have done anything more to show each of us how much we meant to her. I don't think I remember my mom once telling me she loved me. Yet, I never needed her to tell me because I never doubted her love for me. I knew she dedicated her life to me and lived to make me well. She never let me see her cry either. No matter what happened, she was strong. Whenever I would start feeling sorry for myself and whining about things that I didn't want to do, she would tell me, "La vida es un valle de lágrimas. (Life is a valley of tears)." She said that suffering was to be expected because God never promised us a rose garden. She told me time and time again that we had to accept our cruz (cross) with courage. When I was young, I didn't really like or accept her view of life. However, when I became much older, I understood those words. For her, life was a valley of tears, and we, her family, were her only rose garden.

It took me months to get used to my medical care and education. I made up my mind to make the most out of the situation by remembering my mom's words and my dad's hopes. I knew that I couldn't escape and would have to continue going to school no matter how much I hated it. Fortunately, I was starting to learn more and more words, and I was understanding others better. I was also counting down the days to the upcoming summer vacation. My brothers and sisters had started talking about all they wanted to do during vacation. Though I wanted to be a part of their plans, I knew the summer would be different for me. It seemed that the doctors were determined to get me standing. I had just turned seven and still had not stood on my own two feet except for when I was a baby before polio. I couldn't even imagine what that would feel like. It was more others' desire for me than my own.

During the summer, I had another surgery, but this time my hospital stay was not as long. I was still very angry and rude with the doctors and even tried to yell at them in English. I would scream at the doctors and nurses, saying "Shut up!" Those were the only words that I knew sounded bad enough. My surgery was on my right ankle so that it could handle when I stood on it in the future. I wondered why they kept trying to fix my right leg when I knew it was my better one. I couldn't move my left leg at all but could move my right leg a bit. That didn't make any sense to me.

Matilde was still very involved with trying to help my mom. Trying to sound excited, she said, "After they take off the cast and you go to therapy, they are going to measure you for leg braces." I thought to myself, *If it's anything like the braces I've seen, there is nothing to be excited about.* At school I had seen some kids with braces, but they didn't look too comfortable or pretty. I thought to myself, *I would much rather wear my sister's high heels.*

As my ankle recovered, I still had a teacher come and give me lessons, which I thought was unfair because my brothers and sisters didn't have to learn during the summer. Once they removed my cast, I had physical therapy, both at home and in the hospital. At least this time, it didn't hurt as much as after my previous surgery. The doctor scheduled me to go to a different place so that I could be measured for braces. I hoped that I would be missing some school because of these appointments, but sadly, the school bus would take me to the appointment and then bring me right back to school after the appointment. My mom would just meet me there.

The first step to getting measured for braces was something I didn't expect. The doctor came in and he started to wrap me with wet bandages, all the way from my hips to my toes. As he did this, I felt the bandages getting very hot. I also noticed that the bandages were getting hard. It finally clicked, and I realized that they were casting my legs. I had never seen how casts worked before. When my leg and ankle had been casted before, I woke up from my surgery with them. I panicked and for a minute thought that I had been tricked so they could cast both legs this time. I started to whimper and say, "I don't want them. Take them off." The doctor then said, "I will take them off in a few minutes." He told my mom, "We need a mold of her legs so that I can make her braces."

The doctor had told the truth; he did take off my cast with that loud drilling saw. He was extra careful pulling the top off, first from my right leg and then from my left. He then put the mold of my legs to the side and began to measure me as he was writing notes on a notepad. He measured from my hip to my toes, my hip to my knees, and my knees to my toes. He thought out loud and murmured, "Hmmm, her left leg is an inch and a half shorter." He also noticed that my shoe sizes would have to be different. He asked my mom, "What color shoes do you want, white or brown?" I was hoping she would say white, and thankfully she asked me, "Que color quieres?" I quickly responded, "Blancos." I thought white would match with more of my clothes. The doctor had finished all the things he needed to do and scheduled another appointment in two weeks for my first fitting. The attendant told my mom that she would schedule the appointment with the school. The school was involved in all these efforts to "fix me."

CHAPTER 7

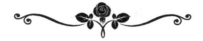

I was starting to feel better about school. Some of the attendants really liked me and were nice to me. I was also starting to make a few friends. But I was more interested in learning English than anything else. One teacher, Ms. Jennings, would have weekly spelling tests and would reward anyone who got all the words right. She took all those who got a hundred percent to the cafeteria and would let us pick out the soda of our choice—though she only gave us fifteen minutes to drink the entire bottle. I always chose a 7UP and gulped it down, not wanting to leave a drop. I drank a lot of 7UPs that year.

I've always considered Ms. Jennings one of my favorite teachers. It wasn't only because of the carbonated drinks I got each week, but because she always commented on my writing and said that someday I would become an author. I wanted to believe her so badly. I was always proud that she would read my paragraphs to the class. These compliments, and Ms. Jennings's encouragement, helped me become more confident in my English. Ms. Jennings was the opposite of my previous teacher, Ms. Parson, who insisted that I spell Pascuala with a *q*. She would put a huge red mark across the *c*, replacing it with a *q*. I couldn't explain to her that I already knew how to write my name and that it *was* with a *c* and not a *q*. I didn't give up; I continued spelling my name the right way. I was glad to get out of her class.

Another reason why I finally began to like school was because of Mr. Berg, my physical therapist. He introduced me to using the pool for therapy. He taught me how to swim without the use of my legs. I was able to float so easily. Though I had never walked on solid ground, he taught me to walk in water. I used my right leg to skip forward. I just used the one leg because my left leg had a mind of its own and always floated away. He was very patient, and when I couldn't do something, he adjusted the exercise so that I could. I felt agile in the water, not dependent and weak like I normally felt. Swimming became my favorite sport because it was the only physical activity I could really do on my own.

I went back and forth to the brace shop, and the braces were coming along nicely. I had tried them a few times, trying to pay attention on how to buckle each of the straps. The doctor wanted to do just a few other adjustments and said that I would have my braces in two weeks. He explained that I had to go to therapy at both the hospital and school to learn how to walk with the braces and crutches.

Unfortunately, the plan didn't work out as the doctor expected. One evening, my mom sat me on the sofa to rest from being on the chair the whole day. She told me she would bring my dinner to me so that I could eat while I watched TV. She brought an aluminum table that was starting to rust so that I could put my plate and drink on it. I found it easier to put the drink on the floor and the plate on my lap. I started to eat and when I bent down to pick up my Kool-Aid, I lost my balance and fell over. My leg twisted in a weird direction and it hurt so much I screamed in pain. Everyone ran to the living room and saw me on the floor. When my mom and sisters attempted to lift me, I cried even louder. My leg really hurt, and I didn't want them to move it or touch it. My mom told my dad to call a cab so she could take me to the hospital.

When at the hospital, my leg was x-rayed, and the pictures showed that I had a fracture on the lower part of my leg. My leg was casted, and I was sent home. The doctor anticipated that I would need the cast for at least six weeks. We didn't get home until almost the next morning. My mom asked Matilde to call the brace shop to cancel the appointment and the school to inform them about my injury. The school told Matilde that they would send the homebound teacher to my house so that I wouldn't fall behind. Standing on my own two feet had to wait a bit longer.

Three weeks after the fracture, my mom took me for a follow-up appointment. She was perplexed about why I had broken my leg when I had just fallen from the sofa. The doctor explained, "Her bones are very weak from the lack of utilization. She has to be careful because any fall could result in a broken bone." Perhaps this changed my attitude about school. I was getting restless being at home all the time; I hated to admit that I even missed my bus ride in the mornings. I also missed talking to the few friends I had.

It took me much more time than the average person would need to recuperate from the broken bone. Again, because of the cast, my leg felt very weak, and I had to have therapy. It wasn't until I turned eight, after my rehabilitation, that I was able to continue with the plan to get me into my braces. I was taught about the braces' knee locks and how to always make sure to lock them before starting to walk. The doctor warned, "If you don't lock your brace, your knee will give out because it's not strong enough. You will fall." The shoes were bright white, and I did notice that one shoe looked smaller than the other. Plus, I noticed that my left shoe had a thicker sole than my right shoe. Not at all shoes that I could show off.

It wasn't until that summer that I got my braces and stood up for the first time. It was not comfortable at all. The metal braces dug into my skin and hurt a lot. They pinched my upper thighs. I felt like a robot and didn't like that my legs had to be straight all the time. I was taken to a therapy room and they stood me at the edge of two long silver bars. The therapist gave me instructions and checked to see if I could understand. When I didn't, she pointed to the leg she wanted me to move. The brace pinched every time I took a step, but I did like being on my feet. I had never felt so tall. With pride, I looked at my mom, and she had the biggest smile I had ever seen.

I am sure she was thinking that all the suffering she had gone through was worth it for this moment. She was so proud. She didn't have a camera, or I'm sure she would've taken pictures. My mom had prayed for this for so long, and now it was real. What everyone told her would be impossible was happening right before her eyes. That weekend, she took me to a professional photography studio so that they could take pictures of me standing. I stood tall, with my red blouse and flowered pants, as the photographer took the picture. My mom held on to me behind the curtains to make sure I didn't fall. She wanted to keep this happiness locked in her memory forever, and this picture helped her do just that. She felt blessed that I was standing, even if she had had to wait for eight years!

Every time I began to feel better, though, something always reminded me of my disability. When the bus came each morning, my mom had to bring me down the stairs. As I was getting older and heavier, my mom felt that it was not safe to bring me down in my wheelchair. She had begun to first bring the wheelchair down and then carry me down afterward. One day, it had snowed at night and the stairs were slick. As she was carrying me, she slipped and fell down all twelve steps. But she protected me and never let me go. The bus driver quickly came over to help. He grabbed me and sat me on my chair and asked my mom if she was OK. Though her pants had ripped as they'd scraped the cement stairs, my mom slowly got up, brushed the snow off, and motioned that it was OK for me to go to school.

No matter what, my mom never let me worry about her well-being, instead pushing me to focus on school and my medical care. As time went on, I became more confident in my knowledge of English. Perhaps I learned it quicker because of so many doctors' appointments. Certainly, all that individualized education from hospital and homebound schooling also helped me to have the undivided attention that helped me learn English much quicker. By fourth grade, I was already able to have conversations in English. I was able to speak for myself and let others know how I felt. For instance, if my brace didn't feel right, I made sure to tell the doctor so that he could adjust it before I went home. Matilde couldn't always go with my mom to my appointments, so I soon became the translator for my mom. By the age of ten or eleven, I was my mom's own personal interpreter during my doctor visits.

By this age, I had already broken my bones at least five times; I didn't know then that I would later have three more breaks. I had close to a dozen surgeries, always on my right leg. Hospitals became part of my life. Regardless of how we got there—whether someone gave us a ride or whether we took a taxi or a couple CTA buses—the hospital was now a familiar place to me. The only part of the road trip I liked was looking at the beautiful lawns of what I eventually learned was DePaul University. I still didn't like staying in the hospitals, but at least I knew what to expect and now could voice my needs and ask questions. I was used to navigating through school and hospitals all alone. Appointments, rather than being something to fear, became just a nuisance. I learned to make the best of my world, be it school or the hospital. I learned that getting angry and revolting didn't change my situation. I had to survive by adjusting to my environment and seeing the best of each place.

Spalding was both an elementary school and a high school. The only thing that separated the primary grades from the high school was a hallway. Although most kids wanted to cross over to the high school and were eager to graduate from elementary school, my goals were different. I was still unhappy that just because of my polio, I had to be segregated away from my family as if something was terribly wrong with me. I wanted to leave the school as soon as possible and join what I considered to be "normal" people. I was counting on my belief that once I graduated from eighth grade, I would be able to go to the same high school my siblings were attending. I felt that if I did my time, and followed the rules, I would someday be able to leave and be with people who were normal. I had no idea that, just a little over a decade later, there would be a law passed called the Americans with Disabilities Act (ADA) that would consider segregation discriminatory.

With time, my attitude began to change. I began to try to understand the people around me. When I saw a kid with a helmet, I had the courage to talk to him even with my limited English, and to my surprise, I found him to be very normal. He wore the helmet for protection because he was prone to having seizures. He stopped being weird once I realized why he was wearing the helmet. Similarly, I decided to approach a kid in my class who was blind. I asked, "Do you need help going to the cafeteria?" It was now time to go to lunch, so I thought I'd volunteer to help. He accepted my help and held on to my wheelchair as we walked towards lunch. A friend of mine named Quinn, who had muscular dystrophy and lacked the strength to lift his arm, always whispered my name for help when his arm slid off the desk while we were taking a test. I discovered that many of the students at Spalding were going through hard times too. Realizing what others dealt with made me feel less sorry for myself.

I'd say that I was bilingual by the age of twelve. I think that is when I had my first dream at night conversing in English. I also started to think in English. My English language skills were helpful to my mom and to me. Having to interpret difficult situations helped me grow up and skip many painful aspects of my childhood by forcing me to separate emotionally from what was happening. For example, during one doctor's appointment, I had to interpret for my mom about a procedure that perhaps a twelve-year-old should be sheltered from hearing. The doctor recommended a surgery based on his examination, and I had to tell my mom all the gory details as if I were talking about someone else. The doctor said, "She needs a surgery to stop her growth since her right leg is now three inches longer than her left. It is getting more difficult to hide the difference in length and if we don't do something, by the time she stops growing, her right leg could be six inches longer than the left." Without processing what that meant for me emotionally, I quickly put on my interpreter hat and said, "Dice que necesito una operacion…"

It was like an out of body experience describing this procedure to my mom. I continued translating what the doctor said, "They are going to make two cuts on my right knee, one on each side of my kneecap, to stop my growth." He continued talking about the procedure, the benefits, and the recovery. He even shared details about the dangers of the surgery and what could go wrong. As I was translating, I avoided any emotions by ignoring that I was talking about myself.

My childhood would have been unbearable if it hadn't been for the most loving family I could ever have, and the good times we had when I was with them. No matter the horrors of my medical care and my struggles at school, I knew I always had a loving family to go home to.

I'd say that through the process of assimilation and the difficulties that resulted from having numerous broken bones and surgeries, I was robbed of my childhood. Shortly after arriving in Chicago I was forced to go through the process of being "fixed." However, I had just as many positive experiences that almost erased all the bad ones. Each of my brothers and sisters always did something to make me feel valuable and loved. For example, my oldest brother Mon, who was the most mischievous member of the family, did anything to make me happy. He once took money that my mom had left on the table to go buy me a toy horse because he knew I'd love it. He got punished and spanked for taking money that didn't belong to him, even when he used it to purchase something for me. How could I not feel special and loved?

My last surgery was to stop my growth, but that was not the last time I had to go to the hospital. As the doctors fixed conditions caused by my polio, others were discovered. I felt that I was like a challenge for any doctor that examined me. It was as if I became a science experiment for doctors to learn more about polio. My mom, not knowing that she could say no, would often approve of me being the "subject" of orthopedic doctors' education. I had to get accustomed to being looked at, so I developed a coping strategy and numbed my real feelings. The hospital never seemed to be done with me.

My active personality helped me survive all of this. I learned to avoid the discomfort of my braces and walked all over the place, ignoring the exhaustion and pain. I had become pretty good at pushing through difficulty so that I could be a part of "life." I would even walk to church several blocks away, and to my Aunt Chuy's house so she could prepare me for my first communion. I couldn't wait until I was ready to walk down the aisle to take the bread and say "Amen." Every Saturday, I would make the walk with one of my sisters who would hang out with my cousin Fidelia while I was taught all about Jesus.

Going to Mass was very important to me. My dad always said, "When you are in Mass, your life stops ticking; so the more you go to Mass, the longer you will live." I wanted to receive the Holy Communion to make sure I would always go to Mass so that I could live a longer life. I am not sure if he just said this to trick us into not complaining about going to church, but his strategy worked. After my first communion, I only missed going to Mass on Sundays when there was a good excuse such as a hospitalization.

I was all over the place and rarely used a wheelchair. The only time I used it would be for very far distances or when the weather was icy. I ignored any discomfort or pain. I had places to go and places to be. I depended on my braces and crutches so much that I would get so frustrated when my brace would break. At times, if it was just a lost screw, my dad would look for one in his toolbox and attempt to fix it. Sometimes we would use duct tape, but depending on the location of the break, it didn't always work. Otherwise, a broken brace would mean that I would be out of commission and back to the chair until the brace could be repaired.

I also had many falls. I would slowly sit up to assess the damage, praying that I didn't have another broken bone. Sometimes, I would count how many times I would fall in a year. I hated that I didn't have the strength to prevent a fall and that any wet spot on the ground could cause my crutch to slip and throw me down. I would joke and say, "Please don't spit or I may slip and fall." Not only did I have to deal with the embarrassment of each fall when everyone would look at me, but I was also still dealing with my brittle bones. Luckily my fractures started to occur farther and farther apart. The braces seemed to protect my bones, and the more I walked, the stronger my bones would get. Although I always knew of the dangers of falling, it never stopped me.

Mama Petra and I had become very close ever since she moved in with us. We were quite the pair. Even with our individual limitations—hers because of her age and mine because of my polio—we were troublemakers. One summer, we decided to walk to the grocery store the next block over. She saw a watermelon and said, "Let's buy one." I said, "No, Mama Petra, I can't carry it with my crutches, and it is too heavy for you." I was trying to be the intelligent one, however she insisted and really wanted the watermelon. We paid for it, and the cashier said it wouldn't fit in a bag, so she just handed it over. Mama Petra held onto it and we left the store. About twenty steps later, she put it on the ground and said, "This is so heavy." I didn't want to be disrespectful by saying "I told you so," so I just smiled and said, "Sorry, but I can't help you." She was so resourceful, though, that when she saw my brother's friend on a bike, she motioned for him to come over. She didn't know English but somehow communicated the problem to him before I could even act as a translator. The boy's bike had a basket on the back, so she slowly lifted the watermelon and put it in the basket, holding onto it because it didn't fit. The concerned boy slowly started to pedal as my grandmother held on to the melon. He tried to go as slow as he could, but it still required my grandmother to trot to keep up. I just stood there watching them, and I laughed until my eyes teared.

Adolescence is a difficult stage of life for everyone, but for me it was even more difficult. I started to pay attention to how different I was and looked. At times, I was rebellious and would go into a pity party, thinking my life sucked, truly buying into my mom's philosophy that life was a valley of tears. How could I not feel sorry for myself when I was the only one in my family who was in the hospital all the time, the only one who broke bones, the only one who had to go to a "special" school. My outgoing personality and my growing faith in Jesus could only do so much for me.

My physical troubles never ended. When I was twelve, my doctor noticed that I had scoliosis (curved spine). He alarmed my mom when he said, "This is the age to correct it or else she will need to have spinal surgery, and that is very dangerous." This was enough to convince my mom. So, he ordered a body brace to go along with my fabulous-looking leg braces. So now, except for my arms, I was going to be wearing braces from neck to toes.

The very day that I went to pick up this newest brace, my mom and I took a cab back home. When we arrived, she helped me out of the taxi and stood me up with my crutches while she paid the driver. Not being used to my new brace that made me feel so stiff, I lost my balance and fell, landing on my left side. The scoliosis brace impacted my arm so hard that I even heard the crack and started to cry in pain. Getting right back into the same cab we'd just gotten out of, off to Children's Memorial Hospital we went. My left arm was casted in a bent position so that I could still try to walk on my braces and crutches. I didn't walk too much, to be honest, and spent most of the time feeling sorry for myself.

Shortly after getting the arm cast off, I was starting to see the light at the end of the tunnel. I had convinced my doctor that I couldn't walk safely with the spine brace, so he agreed to allow me to just sleep with it instead of having it on during the whole day. I must confess that most nights, I took it off, probably in my sleep. I knew this because I would find the brace on the floor in the morning. Luckily, I didn't wake up my two sisters I slept with since they were heavy sleepers.

In addition, with all the pool therapy from Mr. Berg, my right knee had gotten stronger. The doctor decided that I was ready to walk with a shorter brace on my right leg. I would still wear the full brace of my left leg, but at least I could bend my right knee. It is silly, but to me, being able to bend my knee made me feel a bit more attractive, although I despised having to wear two different types of shoes now that I only wore a brace on my left leg.

Throughout these difficult times, my mom kept her strength. Even with all the back and forth to the hospital and caring for the huge family, she decided to bring in extra money by babysitting neighborhood kids. My first nephew, Efrain, Bella's son was born, and she took care of him also. When my nephew began talking, my sister was trying to teach him how to say Mama Virginia. Efrain never got the hang of it, so he made up his own pronunciation and would call her Mama China. That name stuck, so all the other kids, and sometimes the adults, in the neighborhood would call her Mama China too.

Pooling the extra money my mom made from babysitting, managing the money my dad earned, and getting help from my older sisters, my parents kept saving money with the hopes of purchasing their own home. My mom missed the corral in La Purísima; she always loved flowers, but, as renters, we couldn't plant in the yard. With her frugal ways, and with my sister Kika as co-borrower, she finally saved enough money to make a down payment for the purchase of a two-flat with a basement.

CHAPTER 8

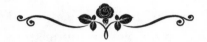

The day we moved to our new home on Parkside, a neighborhood further west but still in Chicago, I was released from the hospital after another bad leg break. My mom had to juggle bringing me home while still moving. One of the first pieces of furniture moved was a reclining seat, which was placed in the living room, ready to receive me when I arrived from the hospital to my new home. When we got there, she sat me on the recliner as she hurried around with the rest of the move. She asked my brother Lalo to run down the street and buy me some food. A Wendy's happened to be around the corner, so Lalo bought me a single cheeseburger. I was still a picky eater from my earlier traumas in the cafeteria at Spalding and had never had a burger. I guess after five years in Chicago, and because I was starving, it was time for me to eat my first burger. I must have liked it because it certainly wasn't my last Wendy's burger.

The new home was great. We all loved it. My mom was excited that she now had a yard that belonged to her. We moved in the fall, but she was eager for spring to arrive; she immediately began to plan what she wanted to plant in the spring. Every year thereafter, she had the most beautiful garden. She took such care of every flower she planted. During planting season, she would go out to tend to her garden at the crack of dawn while we were sleeping. During the day, she would tend to us, to the grandchildren she watched, and to the neighborhood kids that were entrusted to her. Then she would go out to her garden once again in the evenings. She taught both children and adults to respect the flowers, naming them all after one of us or one of her grandchildren. My mom wasn't embarrassed to admit that she talked to the flowers, often saying, "You see those two flowers? I married them." Above all, she taught us not to cut them because they had life. I learned so much about life and the beauty of it from my mom's love and devotion to her garden.

There was so much to like about our new home. First, it meant that my sister Angelita could be closer because she and her husband rented the second floor. Second, I learned that I'd have to go to a different school. There was a closer school, Burbank, that would accept students with disabilities. Unfortunately, I would only be there one year because it was an elementary school that went only to fifth grade. For middle school, I had to go to a brand-new school, Hanson Park, that had just opened for students with and without disabilities. I never expected to leave Spalding before eighth grade. I don't know if I was happy to leave now that I had made up my mind to do as well as I could.

My stay at Burbank School was short since I only went for one year, fifth grade, but I do have a great memory. At Burbank, I encountered the first adult with polio I'd ever met. Ms. Zelesko, whom I'm still in touch with, did one-on-one sessions with students with disabilities to provide extra support per the individualized education plan (IEP). She immediately became my role model. It gave me hope to see that individuals like me with physical disabilities could have successful careers. I met with her every day for one class period and she would help me with vocabulary. What I enjoyed most is that she taught me how to write calligraphy. I loved the different shapes of letters. This skill came in handy for addressing the many invitations for my siblings' weddings. It was so important to see someone who was like me. This motivated me to keep pushing forward.

A year later, once at Hanson Park School, I loved it. I went to Hanson Park for three years—sixth, seventh, and eighth grades. I was starting to dream about boys, and I developed a crush on any cute boy I saw. I also made friends at the school who lived very close to me. I became good friends with Rosanna, who also had polio. She had gotten it in the Philippines and used a wheelchair all the time. I loved her personality and her wild side. She got me involved in things that I never dared to do, like wheelchair square-dancing and even wheelchair modeling. Every Saturday Rosanna's father took us for our "do-si-do and away we go" lessons. We were boy crazy and both of us had crushes on boys who were too busy to even notice us. She was in love with John, and I was in love with Keith. Once, I lied to my parents and told them I'd be at Rosanna's house. Instead, we met the boys at a pizza joint, called Q's Pizza, near our home. It felt so good to be a normal lying teen.

Rosanna and I were the typical immature teenagers. We were both full of dreams and wanted our disabilities not to hold us back. The only time that we ever discussed our polio was when Rosanna suggested we break the "spell" that was cast upon us that caused our disability. She asked me to go to her house so she could perform the ritual that would allow us to walk again. She lived a few blocks away, too far for me to walk there, but my brother or sister would push me in my wheelchair and leave me there for a while and then pick me up. We went into her room, which she had prepared with many lit candles. My heart raced with excitement. Somehow, I really thought that we would walk after we chanted the words she wrote in her notebook. I cannot remember the exact words, but I know I said the chant as Rosanna indicated. But, by the time I was ready to go home, sadly, I was still in my wheelchair. The spell had not been broken. I didn't know it then, but Rosanna would end up being a lifelong friend.

I also hung around with kids on my own block. I found out that a family, who also had immigrated from La Purísima, lived a few houses down. I quickly became friends with Estela, who was around my age. She would come over to my front porch, often with her cousin Maribel, and we would play with a ball or just chit chat while we waited for the ice cream truck. Every day we met outside until it got dark. My brother Lalo also had friends come over to play. Estela, Maribel, and I goofed off, and on one occasion, Maribel and Estela tied Lalo's friend, Dago, to a tree. Over time, Dago also became our friend.

Often while we played ball and tried to do stunts, the ball went into the next yard where a grouchy older couple lived. It was evident that our neighbor was not pleased that we moved onto his quiet block. He had already complained about stepping on his lawn, making too much noise, and going into his yard to fetch our lost ball. My parents had warned us to be careful and not let the ball go over the fence. Well, one breezy day, as we were playing ball, it went to the next yard. Lalo, our hero, jumped over the fence to fetch it, not knowing that my mom was watching through the back window. When my mom saw that Lalo was in the neighbor's yard, she came out and yelled, "Didn't I tell you not to go into that yard?" My brother quickly responded, "I didn't," but he was still standing on the other side. When my mom saw him there, she didn't know if she should laugh or get angry. She chose the latter—we were all in trouble, and mom made us go inside.

I really don't know how my mom and dad handled each of us dealing with our own issues and personalities. And now, the family was getting bigger with grandchildren and my siblings' spouses. Both of my parents instilled strong family values, and we learned to always stay connected. My parents knew exactly what each of us needed. By now, the only ones still at home were Reyna, Lalo, Rique, and I, so weddings were not foreign to me. Both Kika and Mon had married after we moved to the Parkside home, and Reyna and Lalo would marry soon after as well. Mon moved into the basement and Angelita was on the second floor, while all my other siblings found homes nearby. Since mom babysat my nieces and nephews, my siblings would always visit. I grew very close to my nieces and nephews because I practically lived with them.

My nieces and nephews always accepted and even admired me. They would always agree to my ideas. Angelita's kids, Veronica and

Olivia, who lived upstairs, would love to spend time with me. I had them convinced that they were going to be on *Sabado Gigante*, a Spanish variety show that aired every Saturday on the Spanish TV station. I'd prepare them for dance contests so that they would be ready for the audition. They loved to sleep over because I would let them stay up late and play like they were models. I involved all my nieces and nephews in the fun and would prepare Christmas shows for the family by teaching them carols. We would practice for months and then on Christmas, they would show off their hard work. I was also known as the family photographer because my camera was never too far away to capture the good times.

My parents were very wise. They knew about the dangers of the city and worried about our safety, wanting us to never get involved with the wrong influences. My mom was especially strong and wanted to protect my brothers from drugs and gangs because she knew my brothers were at a susceptible age. My parents made the decision that my oldest brother would go to a Catholic school because he was the most rambunctious. They scraped out money to pay the tuition, and my brother Mon would take two buses to go to his high school, St. Michael's. In addition, she personally went with him to find jobs during the summer. They were always present, and this prevented us from deviating from our values. Mon got married soon after graduating from high school at eighteen. No matter what, my parents accepted us as we were.

The only time I ever saw my mom break down was when she received a call from Mexico and was told her older brother, Chano, had been killed by a lightning strike. My uncle and cousin had been farming in La Purísima when a storm arrived. They managed to take shelter, but the lightning went through a window, striking my uncle and flinging my cousin across the barn. When my cousin woke up, he saw that his own father had died. I had never seen my mom cry, much less out loud, in despair like she did when she heard this news. My grandmother was of course also distraught. My mom had to go back to La Purísima to say farewell to a brother she loved so much.

My dad arranged to travel with my mom and grandmother to support them during this difficult time. It was so difficult for Mama Petra to bury her own son.

My older sisters agreed to watch me and the rest of my siblings during my parents' trip. My dad asked his sister, Tia Chuy, to keep an eye on us as well. One day while my parents were away, I was with my sisters. Reyna had just purchased a pair of platform heels that were very "in" at the time. I watched with envy as she showed my sisters the shoes. Oh, how I wanted to wear that type of shoe and not the ugly braces I wore. Later that evening, when no one was watching, I walked over by the shoes. I sat on the bed, took off my braces, and tried on the shoes. Not being too smart, I decided to try and stand on them, but tumbled down and fell, twisting my ankle. I didn't want my sisters to know what I had done so I pulled myself up onto the bed. I pulled the blankets over me, with my ankle still throbbing.

The next day, I woke up and my ankle hurt so much. I tried to put on my brace, but my foot was too swollen, so I got into my wheelchair instead. My sisters, busy doing all the chores, didn't question why I was in my wheelchair. When my Aunt Chuy came to visit later that afternoon, though, she asked me, "Why are you in your wheelchair?" I remembered that she taught me about sin when she was preparing me for first communion, and I knew lying was one. Still, I didn't want to fess up to what had happened, so I fibbed and said, "I'm just tired." She then looked down and saw my left foot and saw how swollen it was. By now, my toes were barely visible, almost as thick as my upper leg. She got on her knees to take a closer look and said, "This does not look right." She asked my sister if she knew why my ankle was so swollen, but my sister was even more shocked. I ended up being taken to the hospital, and upon my mom's return, I was in a cast one more time.

My mom was so alarmed to find me in a cast. She asked me, "What happened?" I didn't have the guts to lie when I looked at her all dressed in black, which she wore for a year because of her brother's death. I saw her with the saddest expression on her face ever. "I fell down," I said. She waited for a few seconds hoping that I would go into detail, but when I didn't, she asked, "How?" I told her what I hadn't shared with my sisters and aunt, saying, "I tried Reyna's shoes and fell." She continued with the interrogation, and this time asked, "Why?" I started to cry and said that it wasn't fair that I couldn't wear nice shoes and had to use the ugly braces. She responded in a way that I will never forget. She said, "At least you have feet to wear shoes. Other people don't have feet and would love to be able to wear your shoes, but they cannot." From then on, I stopped complaining about my ugly shoes.

When I graduated from elementary school, I wanted to apply to go to the high school for smart students, Lane Tech. Several of my classmates were applying to go there. If not, I would be fine going to the high school in my district, Prosser High School. Well, neither of the schools were options for me. The concern was that, in case of an emergency, I would be stuck on the second floor, and they didn't want that liability. To my disappointment, I was told I had to go to Spalding again, this time to the high school side. It felt as if someone had stamped my forehead with a REJECT sign. I felt that, once again, I was being robbed of options. Rosanna's family moved to the suburbs, so she was able to go to a mainstreamed high school. Not only was I going back to Spalding, but I was also losing my only true friend. It was time for another pity party.

CHAPTER 9

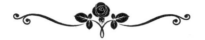

After exhausting any possible way I could go to either Lane Tech or Prosser High Schools, back to Spalding I went. This time, my bus ride was much longer since we were further west after we moved. I would be the first one to be picked up because I was always the person who lived the furthest. I was not too happy with my situation and pouted for a few weeks.

I started reading books to entertain myself during the two-hour commute. Sometimes I couldn't concentrate because this guy would always stare at me. Totally unashamed, he would even wink each time I caught him. He introduced himself as Ray, so I felt the polite thing to do would be to share my name. That was a mistake. He annoyed me with his insistent attempts at conversation. He would ask, "What are you reading? Do you like music? What is your favorite movie?" He would ask question after question and wouldn't get the hint that I was mad and had no interest in making a friend. But his persistence paid off. We ended up becoming friends.

The bus driver, Dwight, and the attendant, Ms. Humphry, made every effort to make the ride fun for us. As the school year progressed, they did things that were totally unexpected. Dwight, as he asked us to call him, announced that, in his bus, "Smoking is permitted— even pot—but you have to open the window." We all looked at each other with puzzled faces. One of the students took his word for it and lit up a joint. I had my mouth open in disbelief and waited to see if Dwight or Ms. Humphry would say something, but they didn't.

Fridays were especially fun. On the ride back home, Dwight would go to different fast-food establishments and buy us all food. His favorite spot was Home Run Inn Pizza. And in the mornings, if he was good with time, sometimes he would buy us donuts. He was not afraid to pull over and hand us all our food. Ms. Humphry would help Ray, who due to a stroke, couldn't use one of his hands. I was fortunate to have Dwight and Ms. Humphry drive me to school all four years. They certainly worked hard not to make us feel "disabled," but simply normal high schoolers.

I started my freshman year with a chip on my shoulder, angry that I was "forced" to go to this school. I didn't realize that my poor attitude just made things more difficult for me. I shut down and didn't allow myself to like anything. I got tired of these feelings, so again, I made the decision to make the best of it. I relaxed and started to make friends, looking for the positive side of things. I told myself, if you can't beat 'em, join 'em. I became very active and joined every possible activity. At the same time, I worked hard academically. I met three very cool teachers—Mr. Keane, a drafting teacher; Ms. Juntunen, a social studies teacher; and Dr. Rosales, a Spanish teacher.

Mr. Keane was very sarcastic and had a dry sense of humor. He was the advisor for the Newspaper Club, of which I was a member. He would come up with the silliest news stories. Once, he took a picture of me dressed up as Colonel Sanders, with a fake white beard and a white scarf to cover my brown hair, after I wrote an article as if I had interviewed the owner of Kentucky Fried Chicken.

Ms. Juntunen was fun in how she taught social studies. In her class, I started to think about what I wanted to be someday. One semester she taught us about courtroom procedures. The class was split into two groups. One group was for the plaintiff, and the other one for the defendant. The case was about a car accident, and we had to play out the situation in a courtroom. I really got into this. I studied the facts in detail and developed a defense that made our team win the case. After this lesson, I started to dream about becoming a lawyer for real. I wanted to change the laws that would make the lives of people with disabilities better.

Ms. Juntunen also encouraged me to enter a writing competition that, if I won, meant I could be selected to go to Washington, DC. She said, "Pascuala, I think you would have a chance in this competition." She handed me the rules and said, "All you have to do is write an essay about what it means to be a citizen." I told her, "But I am not a citizen." She looked at all the requirements and didn't see anything indicating you had to be a US citizen. So, I wrote the essay, figuring I had nothing to lose. Well, I must have convinced the judges, because I was selected to represent Illinois. Ironically, I was probably the only one there who was not a citizen, not to mention the only one with a disability.

My all-expense paid trip to Washington, DC, was amazing. I decided to take my wheelchair because I knew that there would be a lot of walking based on the itinerary. One sophomore from every state went on the trip. We went to all the museums and monuments and even to the White House. Everyone wanted me to feel like part of the group, so they would help me get on the bus and often carried my wheelchair for me. I loved learning about the United States, and this experience motivated me to become a US citizen.

My parents always supported me, even when they were left behind worrying about me. I am sure that they worried for that long week because the only time I hadn't slept at home was when I was in the hospital. Still, they gave me their blessing and let me go. I am so glad they did because experiences like this showed me that life can be beautiful and that we all can experience many happy moments.

The third teacher that I really enjoyed was Dr. Rosales. It was my first time studying Spanish, and to my surprise, I found it very easy, even after only being in school for one week in La Purísima. He gave weekly tests, and if we received an A, he would give us a golden dollar, which he called a "Rosales Dollar." I saved about forty dollars that school year. In all my schooling, I had never had a Hispanic teacher before. I was proud to see a Latino in front of the classroom. When I told him this, he showed me the next paycheck he received. He said, "Someday, you will earn more than this." My mouth dropped since the check was over a thousand dollars. This encouraged me to work hard. Now, a paycheck of a thousand dollars no longer makes my mouth drop.

Dr. Rosales had only one daughter, who was around my age. He invited a few of us from his class to go to his home for dinner and to meet his family. His wife cooked spaghetti for dinner. I had never had spaghetti, but it reminded me of fideo, a noodle soup my mom often made. It was difficult for me to figure out how to eat it until someone showed me how to roll it around the fork. It was delicious. I instantly became an Italian food fan. It was a very special evening because I was able to see how successful people live.

I didn't find school very challenging, except for calculus. I studied calculus one-on-one with the math teacher after he noticed that math came easy for me. He didn't know that I was good only because my older siblings were learning it in school. I took several other classes as independent studies because I'd asked my teachers for subjects that were not being offered. I wanted to learn accounting, so a teacher gave me a book and we worked on it during study periods.

I continued with swimming, but I didn't like that they forced us to use their swimming suits, which were all stretched out and uncomfortable. After changing into our blue, faded swimsuits, an attendant would get us into all-aluminum wheelchairs and push us to the pool area where there was a slide. We would transfer onto the slide and dive in. I hated getting out, because it was much harder to scoot up, especially when I was all wet. Swimming has always been the only exercise that does not tire me out and cause my body aches and pain.

I also played the clarinet in band class. Truthfully, I chose that instrument because I liked how it looked. I have been gifted with many things, but musical talent is not one of them. Still, I joined Ms. Kamp's band. It was obvious that Ms. Kamp's world was all music. She was so unique looking. She had completely white hair, including white eyebrows and white eyelashes. She was an excellent musician. It always impressed me how she was able to pick up on the slightest mistake, which unfortunately was often attributed to me. Still, she encouraged everyone. She pushed us to learn music, focusing most on students lacking musical talent like me. Believe it or not, she even prepared me to play a solo in a national clarinet contest. I played "Yesterday" by the Beatles and placed second. I did practice a lot, so though I lacked musical talent, I was proud to have won a medal.

My family always supported my activities and were glad that I was adjusting and getting involved in school. Whenever possible, my brothers and sisters attended my school-sponsored events. The school was twenty miles away, so it wasn't always possible for them to come. However, they did attend several of my band concerts. I am not sure what impressed them most—listening to the band music or looking around and seeing so many different types of disabilities. Whenever they visited Spalding, they would talk about how lucky I was because my disability wasn't as bad.

Teachers didn't challenge the students much at Spalding. It felt like they didn't have high expectations of us. I think most of the students accepted this and just conformed. Though we were not directly told so, I am sure many teachers thought we would end up collecting Social Security Disability after high school. However, the teachers lit up when I asked to learn harder subjects. They never refused to help me out and went out of their way to teach me what I wanted to learn. I did very well in high school, but how could I do badly when I was competing against myself? I became one of the popular kids, which surprised me because I acted nerdish.

My hospital visits grew further apart. I still walked with a left-leg brace and crutches, but the wheelchair was always my backup. I found it challenging to feel attractive because it was awkward to wear two different types of shoes. I also didn't want to wear dresses because I tried to hide my brace as much as possible. I always wore pants, but after one wear, they would rip because of the brace's knee locks. I learned to put my hand by the holes around my knee because I was embarrassed. My mom tried to find a solution by sewing another layer on the inside, but I didn't like it because it looked bulky.

Between my junior and senior years, for our summer vacation, my parents, Rique, and I went back to La Purísima. Our house in La Purísima was being occupied by my Aunt Fina, my mom's youngest sister who had moved in a few years after we left. We stayed with her and her family. As much as I wanted to remember my past in La Purísima, I couldn't. It felt strange to be there. Somehow, instead of being happy to be back in my birthplace, I became very depressed. I felt that I couldn't do much there. Overall, that trip was memorable, but not for good reasons. Not all the sidewalks were paved, and some were so high. There was running water now, but everything else seemed inaccessible to me. It was ironic that as a child I felt free when I crawled, yet now that I walked, I felt trapped.

My aunt noticed my sadness, so she tried to cheer me up by inviting me to a dance that was taking place one night. Though I rejected her invitation, she didn't take no for an answer. She said, "You have to go. There will be nice-looking guys there." Although I didn't wear much makeup, she insisted on putting some on me. My mom was a bit nervous but trusted that this might be a good experience for me, so she let me go. My aunt and I started to walk toward the hall where the dance would take place. We had only gone a block when one of my crutches got stuck between two rocks, throwing me to the ground. I hit my forehead on the edge of the sidewalk and started to bleed. As always, I had learned to sit and assess the damage to make sure I had not broken anything. Luckily, it was just a terrible bump. My aunt felt so bad and knew we had to go back home. My mom gave my aunt a look but didn't say a word.

Aside from my fall, we had yet another scare. My dad was still struggling with alcoholism. One night, he told my mom that he was going into town to talk to some of the town's men. After several hours, he still wasn't back, and it was already dark outside. My mom said a prayer, as I listened intently to the words. It was a lengthy prayer, but I learned it as we prayed it together multiple times. Dios te salve, reina y madre de misericordia…. Dawn was approaching and our tired eyes were drifting off when we heard a bang on the door. My mom got up quickly to open it. Two men were practically carrying my dad, who was completely soaked in mud. My mom thanked the men and shut the door. She laid my dad in bed and took off his shoes. Struggling, she undressed him and wiped off as much of the mud as she could. She showed me how his wallet had almost disintegrated in the mud, ruining everything in it. My dad was unconscious, so we couldn't even ask him what had happened.

Later in the day, my dad got sick, not just from a hangover, but from the mud he had swallowed. He took a shower and didn't want to talk about what happened. My mom asked him, "Que paso?" and he would respond, "No se." It wasn't until days later that he was calm enough to try to remember what happened. He talked about statues and about his not being able to breathe because he was in a hole. Everything was incoherent, and we couldn't figure out what happened. My mom's best guess was that he was somewhere in the cemetery; it was the only explanation she could come up with. She also tried to figure out who it was that had brought him back to the house, but never did. What happened that day remains a mystery. All that is certain is that the experience scared my dad enough to get him to stop drinking. That was the last time he ever drank alcohol.

I'd hoped to be able to bring some candy back to Chicago that was only available in Mexico, but even that didn't work out. I'd purchased bags of different types of candy and left them on the coffee table in the living room. The front door wasn't totally shut, so my Aunt Fina's pig burst inside, taking the bags of candy with him. So, I can't say the trip ended up being sweet. The two weeks in La Purísima ended up being the last time I ever went back to visit. I returned to Chicago with memories and a new appreciation for all the good things I had.

My senior year went fast because it was fun. I think my group of friends and I had senioritis all year long. It was fun to work on the yearbook since the senior class was the main topic of it. It wasn't a large graduating class like my brother's had been. We only had about fifty students graduating. We did have a prom, though. A bunch of my friends went together as a group, but my partner was Vernon, a soft spoken, African American classmate who used a wheelchair because of his disability. It was easy to convince my parents to let me go because I was on the planning committee and they supported anything that I was involved in. The prom's theme's song was "Up Where We Belong." What I remember most about the prom were my two firsts—my first time getting into a limo and my first time wearing a dress that was so uncomfortable.

Spalding ended up being a place that helped me be successful. Although I don't think it challenged students much, it helped us in other ways. I learned to be my own advocate and to develop leadership skills. I had very supportive teachers who were energized by my enthusiasm and were always happy to help me. At Spalding, I was thought of as one of the brightest students, but I began to doubt my abilities. I had always felt that I didn't fit in at Spalding or with individuals with disabilities, but now I wondered if I would fit in with those *without* disabilities. I wondered if I would be academically disadvantaged when I went to college. I feared not being able to handle the demands. Was I good enough? Was I smart enough? Would I fit in?

My approach was always to push forward even with self-doubts and fears. Even with these insecurities, I knew I had to work hard and leave the rest to God. I took it a day at a time. I knew that my life was unpredictable and that any plans that I made could change in an instant with a simple fall. I continued working from my lists of things to do and hoped that my efforts and strong desire to learn and be successful would get me through. I knew how to be disabled in a school where everyone had a disability. Would I know how to be disabled in a school where I was the only one with a disability? I was starting to figure out my own identity and how disability fit into my own perception of who I was. Since arriving from Mexico, my disability had been something to get rid of; every surgery was to rid me of it as much as possible. But now that I was "as good as it gets," I had to figure out how I felt about my own disability.

I was already figuring out that, culturally, disability was looked at differently. My family always accepted me, but in general, Mexicans viewed individuals with disabilities as those who depend on others, are to be pitied, and are admired for simply getting up. Subtly, I was starting to get the message that I would never live an independent life, never get married, and never have my own family. No one told me that directly, but I sensed that my own culture believed that of me, simply because of my disability. I didn't mind extra care from my immediate family, but it bothered me to think that others pitied me. Sometimes, I would go to Mass and my mom would see someone from La Purísima. They would say things like, "Hay, pobrecita con esos aparatos. (Ay, poor little girl with those braces.)" To survive, I had to start building a shell around me and not let the lack of disability awareness of others keep me from my goals. I was more than the braces, more than the wheelchair, and more than my disability—and I would prove that someday.

CHAPTER 10

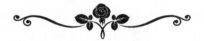

The last few months of my senior year were busy! It seemed that my days under the knife and in plaster were over. I still had many falls but typically without major consequences. I had learned to break the fall with my arms so that the impact wouldn't be so hard. I really began to hate winters because the weather posed a big challenge for me on crutches. Still, I continued pushing through.

In my 1984 graduating class, I was valedictorian, voted as the most likely to succeed, among other similar characteristics. I still had the dream of someday becoming a lawyer to make the lives of people with disabilities better. I also had decided on going to DePaul University after seeing it so many times when I went to Children's Memorial Hospital. In my naivete, I didn't think that my aspirations were unreasonable, but my counselor did.

I made an appointment with my high school counselor. After small talk, she asked, "So what do you plan to do after you graduate?" I said, "Go to college." Although none of my brothers and sisters had gone to college, I knew that my only option was to have a career. My brothers and sisters all had good jobs, but the jobs were in factories, in construction, and at the airport. Plus, my siblings had all gotten married young. None of my sisters finished high school because they started working to help the family. Reyna and Kika later got their GEDs. All my brothers graduated from high school but then started to work. My counselor nodded and said, "I see you live on Parkside.

You belong to Wright Community College." I said, "No. I want to go to DePaul University." She cleared her throat and said, "Oh, that college is very expensive. Let's look at Wright. I know you took typing with Ms. Pope, and you know two languages. I think you would do well as a secretary because it is a sit-down career." I gave her a stern look and once again said, "No. I want to go to DePaul."

The counselor gave me a list of reasons why DePaul wouldn't be realistic for me. She said, "You know, there are no busses that would pick you up." She also said, "You might not get accepted because it is a hard school." In my stubbornness, I said, "If I don't go to DePaul, then I will not go to college." The counselor then said, "Why are you so interested in DePaul?" I thought about telling her the answer she wanted to hear, but I was too angry and instead said, "I want to go because I love their lawns. I have seen them hundreds of times each time I go to Children's Memorial Hospital." I also said, "I want to become a lawyer so that students can go anywhere they want to go to school and not have to come to Spalding." She finally realized that I was not going to change my mind.

I knew I had a list of obstacles ahead of me. I repeated the list in my head over and over: I must apply and get accepted; I must apply for financial aid and find money to go; I must learn to drive to get there. To get started, I had the counselor schedule me to take the ACT. Only a handful of students at Spalding ever took the ACT. I also went to an agency called the Department of Rehabilitation Services (DRS) because they had to evaluate me to see if I would be safe to drive. Once found safe, I registered for a class to learn how to drive with hand controls. The hand controls allowed individuals like me, who cannot use their legs, to drive using their hands. A lever is installed near the steering wheel that connects to the gas pedal and brake. Depending on the direction the control is pressed, it will either accelerate or it will brake. As much as I tried to explain to my parents how I was going to drive, they couldn't comprehend it. My dad said, "Really? You are going to drive with your hands when I cannot even drive with my feet?"

I learned to drive in the winter of my senior year. At first it was scary, but I figured out the hand controls quickly. I started to drive in a huge empty parking lot. Because the lot was not being used, it was unplowed, but my teacher thought it was perfect. He said, "If you learn to drive in the snow, you will be prepared to drive in anything." The instructor agreed that I wouldn't need any other modification since I had no problems with the steering wheel. After a few weeks, he said that I was ready to go take the test.

DRS agreed to pay for the hand controls but told me I would have to buy a car. During the summers, I had worked at Spalding tutoring the kids on the elementary side and had saved my money. In addition, my siblings agreed to chip in so I could buy a used car. My dad and brother went with me to buy it. Obviously, I wouldn't be able to test drive it because of my need for hand controls. I just made sure I could quickly throw my crutches in the back when I got in. My brother test drove the car and we all decided on a brown 1981 Chevy Citation with a hatch back. To me, it was the most beautiful car in the world.

My sister Kika went with me to have the controls installed on a Saturday in April. There weren't many places that installed hand controls; the nearest one we could find was in Elmhurst. We weren't expecting the location to be a private residence with an attached garage that was used for the installations. The mechanic had told me to honk my horn when we got there. Not even a minute later, this man comes rolling out of his home in a wheelchair. We noticed that he had no legs. He said, "The installation will take about thirty minutes. Which hand do you use for the control?" I had to think about it for a minute, then said, "I use my left." I couldn't help wondering if he was the person that was going to install them. I soon found out that he was.

Kika was astonished when the man jumped down from his chair and got on a wooden cart that reminded me of the one I used to get pulled around in when I was a child. He used his hands to move it around the Citation. He then got on the floor of the driver's seat, fitting perfectly in the small space. My sister couldn't stop watching. We heard his tools clank and his electric tool go off and on. At one point, he whistled. He had no problem installing the controls. I was impressed with his agility and how he installed the hand controls. When he was done, I asked, "Did DRS give you the voucher for you to get paid?" He said, "Yes, everything is set." My sister asked, "Can I drive the car even if it has controls? She doesn't have a license yet." He said, "Sure, the controls will not be in the way."

Kika couldn't stop talking about how the man was able to fit right underneath the steering wheel. She said, "I can't complain about anything. Looking at him made me realize that I have no reason to not succeed and work hard." Decades later, Kika still remembered that experience. When she feels doubtful or anxious about anything, she pictures the mechanic whistling while putting in the hand controls.

I was very nervous to go to get my driver's license. I practiced a bit more and then thought, *it's now or never.* Mon took me to the DMV to take my driving test. The instructor that took me out on the road didn't even seem nervous, unlike some people who are afraid of the hand controls. I paid close attention to each of the directions, passing the test on my first try and becoming a legal driver. My mom was so happy that I could drive since she never learned how, and she knew how limiting it was to depend on someone else or on public transportation. It was her preference that I always go with someone. She would say, "What if you get stuck in the snow?" So, every time I would leave, she would give me her blessing and say, "Dios te bendiga. Con cuidado!" (God bless you. Be careful).

The streets of Chicago didn't scare me. I was very good with directions and knew my way around Chicago well. I used my dad's teachings to always know the direction I was going. I also learned the blocks based on the street numbers. For example, I lived at the 5600 block, which was Central. I used to live on the 3600 block, which was Kimball. I also have a pretty good visual memory. I said, "If I have been there, I will never forget how to get there." At first, I just drove on the streets and avoided the highways. However, one time

I got onto Interstate 290 by mistake. I was saying the "Our Father" and holding the steering wheel as if it was going to come off. I was petrified. I saw a police officer on the shoulder, so I decided to pull over behind him. I said, "Hi officer, I got on this highway by mistake. I want to go to Chicago." He said, "you are in Chicago." I said, "I want to go west." He said, "You are heading west." I said, "I want to go to Central." He said, "You are heading to Central." He saw my panicked face, and then said, "Get off on the second exit ahead." From then on, expressways were a breeze, and I soon got rid of any nervousness.

Perhaps because of my many appointments, I had learned to be very organized. I thrived on lists and loved to cross things off as I did them. In that way, I was slowly crossing things off the list that would allow me to go to DePaul. My parents didn't know how to help me. The college process was foreign to everyone in my family. My organization helped me do things step by step. Again, because of my experience with hospitals and always navigating on my own, I learned to ask lots of questions. I was not afraid to ask for help. I became my own self-advocate.

The application to DePaul was more complicated than I thought. I was accepted because I had a great GPA and had done well on the ACT. They didn't know that my competition at Spalding was slim, so I ended up being valedictorian with a perfect 4.0 GPA. There were lots of steps that I didn't understand. Luckily, DRS, who helped me learn how to drive with the hand controls, also agreed to help fund college. I was assigned to Mr. McGraw, who I think should have been retired. He was a sweet man, but with little zest or enthusiasm. I was often the one who directed him. However, he agreed to pay for anything that the Federal Financial Aid wouldn't cover. I applied and qualified for most of the costs, so DHS agreed to pay for the remainder and the cost of books.

My dad took a week's vacation from work so that he could help me during the first week of school. My parents were amazing. Though they constantly feared for my safety, they never stopped me from accomplishing my goals. Neither of my parents drove, so it was understandable that they had concerns about my ability to get around. My dad decided that he would go to school with me so that he could help me with my book bag and get my wheelchair in and out of the trunk in case the classroom was too far for me to walk. I told him it was not necessary, but he insisted. I had no idea what he had in mind or else I would have worked harder in convincing him that it was not necessary.

My goal was to pursue a law degree, so during my orientation, the advisor suggested I pursue a sociology degree since it included the most law classes and would give me a taste of the field. Luckily, it worked in my favor because the entire sociology program was at the Lincoln Park campus and I wouldn't need to go to the Loop campus. Later, I also decided on a minor in philosophy because I figured that critical thinking was crucial for becoming a lawyer.

My first class started at 11:00 AM, so I told my dad that I wanted to head to DePaul at 9:30 AM so that I would have plenty of time to find my class. He said, "OK, let's go so you can wait for the CTA bus." I looked at him, confused. "Dad, I plan to drive there." He said, "I know, but I think until you practice driving more, you should drive behind the CTA bus because they go very slow and you won't feel rushed." I couldn't believe it, so I asked, "Are you serious?" He was serious and had thought about it all night. He planned to go with me and then come home on the bus, returning later when I got out. I told him it was too complicated, but he insisted on his plan. So, I followed the CTA bus from North Avenue to Fullerton, waited for the second bus on Fullerton and then followed it until I got to DePaul. I barely made it in time, but luckily the classroom was right inside the first building, by those beautiful lawns. Fortunately, my dad saw that I was a good driver and let me drive the next day without following the bus. I always wondered how he could assess my driving skills when he didn't even know how to drive himself.

My first class was math. Although the classroom was close, I was glad that I was in my wheelchair because I saw the desks with wheels and wondered how I would sit on the chair safely. The class had about thirty students, but I was the only one in a wheelchair. I sat in the first space I saw where I wouldn't be in the way, which was by the door in the middle of the classroom. It was an odd location for the door, but in the long run it worked in my favor. I took a quick look around and noticed that most of the students were white. This was very different from the makeup of my classes at Spalding. I did see a couple with darker hair, but I wasn't certain if they were Latino because I only saw the backs of their heads. The professor went over the syllabus and told us about all his expectations and when the tests were going to be.

CHAPTER 11

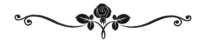

After math class on my first day of class, a nice-looking Latino guy approached me to say hello. He introduced himself as Gerardo. I introduced myself and then kept rolling, mostly out of nervousness and not wanting to be in the way. Gerardo was the first person I met, not knowing that he would be a lifelong friend. He was the first one to show me that I was more than the wheels I was on or the braces I wore—I was a determined person with goals, values, and a strong work ethic, and quite simply worthy of being known. I learned to determine when someone felt comfortable with me and my disability by picking up subtle hints. I recognized immediately that Gerardo was very comfortable around me and that he enjoyed my company.

I was so fortunate to have met so many great friends at DePaul, most of whom were Latino. We had our territory in the main building in Lincoln Park. A common area where students gathered was called The Pit. I believe it was named The Pit because it was sunken into the middle of the building when you first came in. There were stairs to get to the bottom of The Pit with seats all around. Obviously, I rarely went down to The Pit because of the stairs, but in between or after classes, I would sit on a sofa outside The Pit. Gerardo would often see me sitting and would come by and chat. Shortly after, other Latinos saw us, and they too would come to talk to us. Before we knew it, over a dozen friends would meet there every day. I noticed that if someone else was sitting on the sofa and saw us starting to congregate, they would move as if saying, "This spot is owned by the Latinos."

Academics were still my priority, and people knew it. In fact, they appreciated it. My work ethic helped me tremendously because I knew I had something to offer. I would always be willing to revise a paper or to help with an assignment. In return, I wasn't embarrassed to say, "Can you help me clear the snow off my car?" Sometimes when the handicapped parking space was taken, one of my friends would go park the car and then bring it back around for me when I needed it. There was a great give-and-take arrangement between all of us. I was doing well in school, but it didn't come easy. My organization and lack of procrastination were assets. Faculty would assign a paper or assignment, and I would start it even if it wasn't due until a few weeks later. It felt good being successful in competing with my peers, and that I was even doing better than some. My polio had nothing to do with my intelligence, which I'd feared because of my lack of confidence.

Joining a student organization, Latinos Unidos, helped me tremendously with my self-esteem. I met so many students who had the same challenges I did in terms of family, finances, and lack of opportunities. They helped me realize that my disability was not the only obstacle for me. Another real obstacle was my race and people assuming that I didn't belong in positions of power or success. This was very enlightening to me, because for the first time, I stopped focusing solely on my disability and began to feel pride in my roots and heritage. For the first time, I could say that I was proud to be a Latina in the United States.

I studied hard, leaving my house early and not coming home until dark. Besides The Pit, I was constantly in the library. I met one of my friends there, Lucino. Lucino had immigrated from Mexico as a teenager and was eager to learn and grow. Like me, he was often at the library trying to study. He had heard that I was good with writing, so he asked me to revise his papers. After becoming friends,

I would offer him a ride to his house, especially when it was dark. Each time, he had me leave him at the corner, no matter how much I insisted I could take him all the way home. After he learned to trust me, he admitted that he was embarrassed to show me where he lived. I shared some of my own history, and from then on, we realized that we were more alike than different. Lucino is now a successful businessman who has come a long way from the person who had issues showing me where he lived and needing help revising his papers.

Another student that I met through my love for writing was Luis. Luis was a newer immigrant from Mexico who, like Lucino, was learning English. He approached me for help with his papers. Through our interactions, I learned that my family was not as big as I had thought. Luis had nineteen siblings from the same mom and dad. He was attending seminary school while attending DePaul. He was certain that he wanted to be a priest. I used to tell him, "Como creo que en vez de papa, vas a ser camote." I loved teasing him, insinuating that there was no way he would become a priest. He proved me wrong. He is a priest and has helped me on several occasions to celebrate Mass for my family. We remain friends and at times I go to the parish where he is the pastor.

Sometimes my first encounters with people who would become lifelong friends were casual and unplanned. One day while hanging out by The Pit, a person I had not seen before sat right next to me and began talking. He introduced himself as Daniel. I connected immediately with him, not knowing why the affinity I felt was so strong. We became instant friends and we would look for each other any time we were on campus. Just like Gerardo, I felt that Daniel didn't even notice my disability. He had an outgoing personality and he made everyone, including me, feel appreciated. No matter what worries I had, they disappeared when I hung out with Daniel.

I met many other Latino students during my four years of college. I felt valued, and my disability wasn't an issue. Although I was a commuter, like many of my friends, I was very much a part of the social life of the campus. I would go to the Latinos Unidos meetings and attended any of their events. My parents were still strict, but I think I got away with more things than my sisters ever did. Still, they imposed curfews on me. I would often complain saying, "It isn't fair that I have to be home at eleven. Usually eleven is when the party first starts getting good." They would say, "Since you will miss the party, then don't go at all." I would just grunt and start getting ready.

There were a couple of events that remain very vivid memories for me. One was a dance that took place in the gym where the Blue Demons basketball team played. The Blue Demons were doing very well during my time at DePaul. The dance was being sponsored by Latinos Unidos. They had a DJ playing popular music of the 80s. I loved to dance. At home, I would see my sisters dancing their cumbias, and in my mind, I was dancing right along with them. Of course, I had never dared to dance live; it was all in my head. I loved pop music from Michael Jackson, Madonna, Duran Duran, Cyndi Lauper—the list goes on. It had only been a couple of years before college that I had taken down my favorite musicians' posters from my walls.

At the dance, my friends put a few tables together where all of us could sit. They already knew that I wanted to be up front so I could watch people dancing. Daniel said, "Let's all go dance." I looked at everyone, as if his invitation didn't include me. He said, "Yes, you too." I guess I felt so comfortable with my friends that he didn't have to ask twice. We all went to the dance floor. Even on my crutches, I outlasted everyone. The only one that kept dancing was Daniel, who danced with me until the DJ stopped playing. While on the dance floor, I felt so alive. All the previous suffering throughout my life had dissolved. I was free. From that night forward, I never sat out any dance, not caring what anyone might think if they saw me dancing.

That summer, a group of seven of us from Latinos Unidos went to the Wisconsin State Fair. Now that I had a taste for dancing, I wanted more. In the evening, we went to a bar called Marilyn Monroe (who could forget a name like that?). We went during karaoke night, and whoever participated got a copy of their performance on a VHS tape.

Of course, we didn't want to pass on this opportunity and decided to participate as a group. When we looked at the list of songs, the only song we all sort of knew was "La Bamba." We started to sing, dancing to the song, while I used my crutch to simulate a guitar and Daniel pretended to be drinking a Corona. We certainly knew how to act the part, but we sounded terrible, until the shyest of us all, Javier, decided to rescue us with his nice voice. It was so much fun. I wish I had transferred the VHS onto a DVD, so I'd be able to watch it.

Besides dancing, we did other fun things. One day, I wanted to go swimming, and Daniel convinced me to go to the school's pool. I doubted that the swimming pool would be accessible for me to get in, but I figured, with Daniel's help, I would manage. After taking my brace off and changing in the locker room, I went to the swimming pool in my chair. Rick, who I knew hung out with Gerardo, was already in the pool since he swam regularly. I had no problems getting in; I basically jumped in from my wheelchair. We played a few "hold your breath" games and swam for thirty minutes.

After spending some time in the pool, I was ready to get out. I tried using the steps of the pool and my arm strength to get out, but I wasn't succeeding. I tried a bunch of different ways and finally had to admit that I needed help. Daniel, in his usual cheery mood, at first thought I was joking, but when I said, "Oh no, I'm stuck," he realized I was serious. Daniel knew he wouldn't be able to pull me out alone, so he called Rick out of the pool and asked if he could help me. They looked at each other and said, "We can pull you out. Don't worry." Well, I was worried! From outside the pool, they each took one side and started pulling me from my underarms. I groaned and said, "This isn't gonna work." Rick started to get notably anxious and began to pace back and forth. When I saw his reaction, I was more worried for him than for myself. Then, without expecting it, Rick dove into the pool. Daniel and I were in shock. When his head came out of the water, he said, "I needed that!" He then said to Daniel, "I can push her up while you pull her." Rick hesitated, being unsure where to hold me. He was so nervous that he said, "Hold on, I'll be right back." He then got out of the pool again. I wondered where he was going when suddenly he dove into the water once more. When he came up, he said, "OK, let's do it." Both he and Daniel were able to get me out, but I think Rick needed therapy afterward.

With the many experiences we shared, Gerardo and I became the best of friends. He had a part-time job at a nearby shoe store, Father and Son's, and he would invite me to go study with him while he worked. At Father and Son's, I met his brother Jaime. From then on, the pair were my twin towers since they were so tall while I only measured five feet. Their workplace was not always the best place to study. It never failed—each time we would begin, a man would come in to try on shoes. I started to learn all about shoe styles from observing Gerardo work. It was a good diversion for me to get off campus yet still try to get some studying done. One day, on our way out of the shoe store, I tripped on something and fell. Before Gerardo had a moment to panic, he started to sing, "If you are happy and you know it, kiss the ground." I didn't know if I should laugh or cry. I looked up and appreciated how he made the embarrassing moment humorous. I felt completely safe to be myself with Gerardo.

Once, Gerardo invited me over to dinner at his house. I was nervous to meet his parents, but I accepted his invitation. Slowly I climbed the stairs to get into his house. Immediately I felt his home to be serene and warm. His mom and dad welcomed me to their home and invited me to sit at the dinner table. I have always been a picky eater so I was hoping that I wouldn't do anything to embarrass myself. His mom had cooked milanesa de pollo (breaded chicken). When I asked what it was, they couldn't believe it, since it's a common dish at a Mexican table. I had never eaten breaded chicken before but wished I had been introduced to it long before. It was delicious and I instantly became a fan. Of course, Gerardo had already discovered that I wasn't always willing to try new foods, though he always tried to convince me. This time, no convincing was needed because his mom was an excellent cook and the milanesa was tasty.

I also developed a friendship with Jaime, Gerardo's brother, as I got to know the brothers better. These brothers had a way of making any difficult situation lighter by using their humor. On another occasion when I was walking with Jaime on a very windy day, I slipped and fell. The wind practically knocked me down. Jaime said, "Pascuala, you are rolling away. Hold on." Talk about timing; Jaime noticed that Channel 2's news reporter, Harry Porterfield, was nearby doing his weekly "Thumbs-up Chicago" report. I don't know if he signaled him to come over, but the next thing I knew, I was sitting on the ground, giving my "thumbs-up" with a tearful smile. I was on the news that evening.

One of my falls during my college years did have more serious consequences. When I was in my second year at DePaul, two weeks before the end of the spring semester, I was getting ready to go to school and fell. I wish I could say that I fell while doing something heroic or fun, like skiing. Unfortunately, I fell while I was brushing my teeth. I lost my balance while standing by the sink and fell sideways, hitting my right knee directly and forcefully on the bathtub. It was the worst break ever. There was no question that the break was bad because the bone was visible through the skin. I hadn't broken a bone for a few years, so I was not ready for another one, much less for the worst break ever.

The first thing I thought about was school. I was getting ready for finals and had a major research paper due for English Composition II. When I went to the hospital, my right leg was casted from my toes to my thigh. There would be no way for me to attend classes to finish my semester because I had to keep the leg elevated not to mention I had no transportation that could accommodate my new situation. I contacted my friends and professors to strategize how to successfully complete the semester. Luckily, in all my classes except English, I was ahead enough that even without the final, I would still get an A. For English, I just had to turn in the final research paper. I spent the first week after my injury with a Smith Corona typewriter between my legs, typing my paper on the topic of Luther's revolt against the

Catholic church. One of my classmates did me the favor of coming to pick up the paper and turning it in.

After the panic of turning in my paper, I became very angry and depressed, perhaps because I had thought I was done with broken bones. For two months, I was in bed, with my leg elevated, watching the same two movies repeatedly. I watched *Footloose* and *Greystoke: The Legend of Tarzan, Lord of the Apes* over and over on TV. I must have watched each movie at least twenty times. I even memorized the lines. I also took out my anger on my own hair. Because I had long hair, and it was difficult to have it washed while my leg was casted, I grabbed a pair of scissors and cut my own hair short. It was a difficult summer, but as I so often do, I pushed through and continued with my life. I learned that staying in pity parties too long does not work.

Similar to my relationship with Gerardo, my friendship with Daniel grew stronger each year. A while later, I discovered that he was also from La Purísima. Apparently, he had known we shared this in common all along and thought that I knew too. Now it was obvious why I felt so connected and comfortable with him. Daniel was living with a few other guys and a priest in "Casa Claret." I understood Casa Claret to be a place for young men to decide about their vocation for priesthood while attending college. Though Casa Claret was for men, I became a frequent visitor. I often ate dinner with the whole group. Everyone accepted me immediately. One time during the winter, I had gone to dinner at Casa Claret and was not expecting a blizzard to cover the city within hours. I was about fifteen miles away from my home, and what would normally take me 40 minutes to drive, ended up being five hours that night.

As I look back, I have an even greater appreciation for what my parents did for me. They must have worried so much, but they never let their worry stop me from living my life to the fullest. Even on the worst snowy days, my mom would give me her blessing, help me to the car, and just pray that God would protect me. I didn't always abide by their requests to come home at a specific time—sometimes because I would lose track of the hour and sometimes because there was a legitimate reason. When I arrived late at night, I would find my dad, usually in his boxers, standing in the kitchen having a snack, or at least that is what he wanted me to believe. I would try to enter the house quietly, but in case I didn't see him, he would cough or make a noise with his dishes. However, he never said anything, and neither did I. After this happened many times, I realized that he was not having a midnight snack, but rather was waiting for me to get home safely.

My family always looked out for me. At night when I was still studying, my brother Lalo, who worked at the airport until 11 PM, would come in to chat with me. We chatted about his girlfriend Irene, who would later become his wife, and he enjoyed listening to my stories too. We talked while we ate whatever fast food he'd picked up for us on his way home from work. We built a close relationship, and because of these nocturnal chats, I probably gained a few pounds too.

Besides my family life, academics, and my social life, I also balanced part-time jobs. Most of the time, I worked on campus. I worked as a writing tutor during my first semester at DePaul. The Writing Center then recommended me to work for a special program called STEP. STEP was a Saturday program for high schoolers that offered them the first "step" to encourage them to consider college as an option. The students took writing, reading, and math while learning about college life. I really enjoyed the program, and especially appreciated knowing the coordinator, Dr. Rafaela. She was the second Latina I had met working in the field of education. She became a mentor and someone who supported me throughout my college experience.

In my sociology major, I also met friends that I would see in several classes. Shirley, Sara, and Jenna became good friends of mine. I met Shirley in my only job off campus. I was a tutor for Kelvyn Park High School students that struggled with English as their second language. It was ironic that the same school that would have rejected me as a student now hired me as one of their employees. (One of the students I tutored was Aureliano, who later became a very successful television news reporter on a Spanish TV channel.) Shirley and I worked together, and I soon found out that she didn't live far from me. She was taking the CTA bus, so I offered her a ride instead.

Shirley is also now a lifelong friend because we shared so many experiences. Although I met Shirley at Kelvyn Park High School, we also ended up taking many classes together at DePaul. We also began to coordinate our schedules so that I could drive her to school. I became not only her driver, but my other friends' driver as well. I became the unofficial DePaul University limo with a tune from Los Bukis, my favorite Mexican music group, always playing. In the morning, I would first pick up Shirley at Central and Fullerton, then drive east on Fullerton to pick up Gerardo and his brother Jaime, then drive a few blocks further east and pick up Miguel. I didn't mind picking everyone up, but I did mind that Gerardo and Jaime were rarely ready when I got there. I would honk the horn and usually wait at least fifteen minutes for them to come out. Much later, Gerardo admitted to me that sometimes they would hear the horn and quickly jump into the shower because they knew I was getting impatient.

Shirley and I also worked another job together. We both decided to work for DePaul's call center where students would call alumni to ask for donations. The job was every evening for four hours, from five to nine. During our break, we would run to Domino's and eat an entire medium pizza during our allotted 30-minute dinner break. We tried having fun during this stress-filled job, but sometimes it wasn't possible. We called alumni and started off by asking for a million-dollar donation to be in the President's Club. We had a script that we couldn't deviate from, even when we knew that we would get a lot of hang-ups from people when asking for a million dollars. Shirley and I would sit next to each other, which often ended up being a mistake. Our giggles were uncontrollable at times, but how could I control myself when I heard Shirley saying, "Hello, Mr. Hurley, this is Shirley"?

Sara was someone whom I believed would be a lifelong friend, but I lost track of her due to life circumstances. Sara was a beautiful Puerto Rican girl who thought she wanted to be a nurse but later switched to sociology as her major. She was so pretty that she was even a contestant for the Miss Illinois pageant. We took many classes together, but I still wondered why she would want to be friends with a girl like me. Shirley, Sara, and I often went out on the weekends. Sometimes we went to the movies or out to eat at our favorite locations, Mr. Subs or Bakers Square, and on rare occasions, we went to a nightclub.

I remember when we went to a nightclub that clearly showed me how men prefer beauty over any other quality. Sara, perhaps because she knew she was pretty, would often give guys the cold shoulder. When we went to a nightclub, she wouldn't even give any guy the time of day. Sometimes I even felt embarrassed for how she treated them. I, on the other hand, was always friendly with anyone. When guys approached us, I'd smile and chat with them. That night, a guy in his twenties came by and began talking to the three of us. Sara was clearly not interested, Shirley was cordial, but I was very friendly and joked with him.

The man and I hit it off, chatting, laughing, and having a good time. He even bought us all a round of drinks. He started to share information about himself and felt comfortable talking to me. All the while, Sara was even intentionally showing her lack of interest to the point of being rude. When it was time to go, we started to gather our things and I said farewell. The man, who had talked to me all night, and who had been ignored and rejected by Sara, said, "Sara, can I have your phone number?" Sara rolled her eyes and rudely got up without responding. Shirley and I got up and said good night.

While driving home, I couldn't help but start to feel sorry for myself. After I dropped them off, the flow of tears couldn't be stopped. I asked myself, *how come life is so hard?* I couldn't understand why. I was the one who talked to the guy and was the one who made him laugh, yet he preferred the person who was so mean, rude, and disrespectful. I knew the answer to the question I was asking. Sara was a beautiful girl, and I wasn't. I was only good enough to be a friend. I was someone to talk to but never someone to love. I was the one who heard all about the relationship woes but never the one in a relationship. And the only reason for this was because of my destiny to have polio. I didn't tell anyone, but that weekend, I started another pity party. As I often did when that type of heaviness entered my heart, I just pushed harder and looked for another goal to numb me so that I wouldn't hurt as much.

Sara was not to blame for how society viewed what was important. She was a very nice person, and sometimes I saw that even with her beauty, she had her own demons. She wasn't a very confident person, and unlike me, she struggled trying to figure out what she wanted to do. We were about to finish our degrees when Sara decided to apply to American Airlines to be a flight attendant. She got an interview at the headquarters in Dallas, Texas. She begged me to go with her, promising to pay all my expenses. Somehow, I convinced my parents to let me go, and we flew to Dallas.

We had a good time during our four-day stay in Texas, even if it just turned out to be a mini-vacation because Sara, again, changed her mind and didn't go to the interview. Her lack of confidence must have gotten the best of her. I really got to know Sara during that trip, and I began to realize that sometimes that which we envy is no better than what we have. She and I became excellent friends, so much so that I went on my first cruise ever to the Caribbean with her that summer. Again, my parents let me go, though I am certain it was not easy for them to do so, knowing that I would be in the middle of the ocean somewhere. My parents' courage allowed me to participate in the unknown and helped me grow to understand the world.

Cruising became my preferred form of vacationing. I hadn't vacationed much other than in the summer spending time at a campground with my family. It was great, though, because access was already there. I loved waking up to new sites, and the enormous ocean helped me to put my feelings into perspective. I had been giving myself too much importance. I was just a speck in the world in the great scheme of life. I learned that God had created me, the tiny speck, with the same love as the gigantic ocean. It was very enlightening.

The cruise was also a lot of fun. I didn't care to go sit out in the sun. I did struggle to get onto the low beach chairs, but there was always a stranger that was willing to give me a helping hand. Sunbathing on the deck was not possible for me because the long stocking under my heavy brace covered my entire leg. I didn't want to tan only one leg, leaving the left one as pale as paper. Still, I enjoyed sitting and watching the activities on deck. Sara was often a magnet for attention, which forced her into playing multiple games. In one, she had to vote for the man with the hairiest chest among ten grizzled-looking men.

My friend Jenna was a different type of friend. Her parents had immigrated from Italy; if I'd thought *my* parents were strict, that all changed after meeting hers. When I visited her once, I was amazed by her living room. The sofas were all covered in plastic. The carpet had been vacuumed with lines going in the same direction. It was obvious that the room was a "living room" in name only. Jenna was extremely anxious and competitive. She always worked to be the top student, to the point of making herself sick. She wanted to go to law school too, so, rightfully so, she worked very hard. She was my focused friend who always pushed me to do better. She got annoyed when she would spend hours on an assignment and I would finish in half the time, yet we would still earn the same grade. We had plans to apply to the same law school and become roommates.

Perhaps because of my strong sense of justice, I met with college officials to talk about the lack of access at DePaul. The college lacked ramps, handicapped parking, and other such things. I figured, if I was going to be a lawyer, why not start advocating for changes that could make lives better for me and future students with disabilities? When I talked to a student life staff member, I noticed that she was not prepared to respond to the list of questions I had. For example, I asked, "Do people with disabilities pay less tuition since we cannot utilize the entire campus due to lack of access?" After advocating for the access, I started to notice ramps where previously there had been a barrier.

I managed to balance a full life. My family became accustomed to my absence during the weekends. Everyone was busy growing their own families; my sisters and brothers began to have children of their own. I viewed my nieces and nephews as my own because I never dared to entertain the thought of having my own family. Though I was getting ready to graduate with my bachelor's degree, I never imagined ever marrying. Culturally, I had been taught about the role of the woman, and I didn't fit that image. I would ask myself, *who would want to marry me?*

I have always felt that my college experience was one of the best times in my life, except for my last year, which proved to be very difficult for various reasons. I was succeeding academically while maintaining different circles of friends, and I didn't want to leave school. I felt connected with so many friends, although at times I would also feel lonely. I worked hard not to allow those thoughts into my mind. Instead, like a good racehorse, I put on blinders to keep the target in focus—success. I believed that by continuing to strive and work hard, my void would someday be filled. Sometimes it worked, but other times, the void got even bigger.

Aside from the stress of figuring the next step in my career goals, this was the first time that I had ever experienced seeing someone die. Mama Petra's health had been deteriorating because of her uncontrolled diabetes. She was admitted to the hospital and passed away while other family members and I were with her. It was hard to watch my mom say goodbye to her mother. It was unreal for me to watch how, one minute, Mama Petra was alive and the next she was gone. I really loved my grandmother, and it was difficult for me to watch her go. My mom took Mama Petra to La Purísima to bury her next to her son. The burial took place on Mexican Mother's Day, May 10. This date brought my mother sadness for many years.

The last year of college was dreadful for me because of the loss of my grandmother and preparing for the possibility of moving out on my own to attend law school. I now had to figure out how to resolve a whole new set of obstacles. I also dreaded having to figure out access all over again somewhere new. Still, I knew I wanted to continue with my goal—I had passed by DePaul University on my way to Children's Memorial Hospital too many times, dreaming of the day I would be on that campus preparing to be a successful lawyer. Besides attending my last classes, I was busy preparing to apply for law school. I couldn't afford the Law School Admission Test (LSAT) preparatory course that Jenna was taking, but I spent a lot of time going over different logical equations. When it was time to take the LSAT, I wasn't too confident but thought that I would do the best I could.

My hope was that my LSAT score, coupled with my above 3.5 GPA, would be enough for me to be accepted into a good law school. I decided to apply to DePaul's law school and to Drake University in Iowa because of its lower cost. Jenna also applied to the same two schools, and we still talked about being roommates. We were both so excited when we received notice that we were accepted to Drake University. I was offered a full ride toward tuition and fees, but I was responsible for paying for room and board. I still thought this was a good deal since I figured I could get student loans. DRS wouldn't fund school past my bachelor's degree. DePaul University also accepted me and gave me a good scholarship, but I would end up paying about the same as Drake if I continued living at home. Since Jenna had not heard from DePaul, I decided to go ahead with my plans to go to Drake University.

The thought of moving out of state scared me. My brother Mon drove me to Iowa to look at the university. I was surprised by how different it was. I didn't really feel connected to the campus, but I hoped that I would get used to it. Jenna and I continued with our plans. We made a list of the items we would need and decided who would buy which items. Our graduation came, and I decided not to attend because it was at the Auditorium Theatre and I feared a lack of access. And sure enough, when I called Student Affairs, they told me I couldn't be accommodated. But I figured that when I became a lawyer, then I would *really* celebrate and would attend that graduation. Many of my Latino friends were still not ready to graduate because they'd been attending part time due to the costs.

Jenna and I planned to move in the middle of August. We had a couple of months to prepare. I was also trying to prepare my parents for this move. I knew they wouldn't stop me, but I also knew they worried about me. I pretended to be strong, but deep down, I was apprehensive. Although I was very independent, my family had always been there to help me. When I couldn't do something, my father would try to figure out how I could, or someone else would step in. They let me do things for myself, but I was not accustomed to struggling, because they were always there. For example, I was in my twenties and my mom still did my laundry. It wasn't because I didn't know how to do it or because I was lazy, but because the space and type of washing machine we had were inaccessible. Likewise, I did go shopping for groceries with my family, but the full responsibility was not mine. In a dorm, I would be the one responsible for the shopping. I worried what I would do away from home.

Cooking, though, was not one of my worries since I always enjoyed preparing meals with my mom. At the time, I didn't always appreciate being in the kitchen with her. Still, I learned how to cook most of her dishes. My mom cooked by intuition and not by recipe. Anytime that I brought to an event a dish cooked with my mom's help, someone would inevitably ask for the recipe. When I told them, "She didn't follow a recipe," they would joke and say, "You just don't want to share it." I was known to cook spectacular chiles rellenos (stuffed peppers). I never enjoyed cooking tortillas de harina (flour tortillas) perhaps because I wasn't a big fan of them and perhaps because I figured it was easier to buy them at the Mexican grocery store. I did know that cooking in a dorm would be limited, so I tried to think of dishes that I could cook using a microwave.

I of course wondered about access at Drake. At DePaul, many of my friends helped me. Even the security guards got to know me, and they suggested where I could park even if it was not an official space. At times, I would call one of them to bring me my car, especially when I had parked far away. Now, I had to rebuild all these relationships so that I could be assisted. I would have to continue to fight and demand access if I wasn't able to get to an area where I needed to go. In the late 80s, there was still no law to require colleges to provide access to students, especially at private universities. Individuals with disabilities like me had to figure it all out on our own.

Just three weeks before our scheduled move to Iowa, I received a letter from DePaul. I opened it, not knowing what it could be. It was a letter informing me that I had been selected for a fellowship to attend the Law School. It included all tuition, fees, and books and even offered an $880 a month stipend for living expenses. At first, I was ecstatic and couldn't believe it. Then, I was in turmoil. What was I going to do? How would I tell Jenna? Maybe she got one too? My family was so happy and proud of me. They had no doubt that the best thing for me was to accept the fellowship that would allow me to continue living at home.

CHAPTER 12

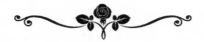

The question that kept going in circles in my mind was, *is DePaul or is Drake in my destiny?* The first thing that I had to do was to find out if Jenna also received a letter from DePaul. After telling my family, I picked up the phone and dialed Jenna's number. The phone rang a couple of times before Jenna's brother picked it up. I said, "Hi Peter, is Jenna there?" He didn't respond to me, but I heard him yelling, "Jenna, it's your friend Paula." He was never able to pronounce my name. When Jenna came to the phone she said, "Hello, Pascuala. What's up?" I said, "I am just calling to see if you received any mail from DePaul today?" She said, "No, I didn't. Why? Did you?" I wanted to kick myself for calling her without being ready to answer her question. I said, "Yes, I did." Jenna waited to see if I would start talking again, but after a few seconds of silence she said, "What do they want?" I tried to tell her in the gentlest terms that I had been offered a fellowship. But is there a gentle way to tell a friend that you can no longer be her roommate? How could I explain that I couldn't turn down an opportunity that makes better sense financially and access-wise? Jenna became quiet and didn't say anything. She cleared her throat and said, "Hey, I was busy doing something. Can we talk later?" I said, "Of course," and then we hung up the phone.

The following days were filled with guilt. I felt that I had made a commitment to a friend and had disappointed her. However, I knew that the best option for me was DePaul. First, I had my family that could and would always be there to help me. Second, I also counted on my many friends. A lot of them were going to the downtown campus already; Gerardo was a business major and would have to take many classes downtown. Third, I wouldn't need to work because the stipend could help me with my expenses for gas and food on campus. On my pros and cons list, DePaul would clearly win. Everything would have been so perfect if Jenna had received the same letter. I also started to feel funny, wondering if I was given this opportunity because of being a disabled Latina woman. And if so, should I accept the offer? In many past experiences, my race and disability had been a disadvantage for me. Should I feel bad now if it was an advantage? So many questions clouded my mind, putting a damper on what should have been happy and exciting news.

A couple of times, I called Jenna and asked if I could go over to her house, but she always had a reason for why it wasn't possible. We both started law school, Jenna at Drake and I at DePaul. My heart ached because I didn't want our friendship to end, yet I totally understood how she felt. I also hoped that in time, she would understand why I had to make the decision I did. I tried to prepare myself mentally so that I could handle the multitude of new obstacles, even with staying at home.

The first obstacle, and probably the most difficult, was transportation. There was no public transportation that was accessible for wheelchair users. My only option would be to drive to Jackson Boulevard and pay for parking. I was shocked at the cost, but I couldn't park in the garage, since the nearest one was about five blocks away, which was way too far for me to walk, especially during the winter. There were some metered spaces which could be closer, but they were taken about 95 percent of the time, so I didn't want to depend on them. I asked the law school for assistance in finding a solution, but they just pointed me to the parking garage. My only option was to park illegally. Because I had handicapped license plates, I read that my car couldn't be towed unless it posed a fire hazard or it obstructed traffic or private property. I also read that I didn't have to abide by any city ordinance that imposed a parking time limitation. For example, if there was a space that said no parking after 2 PM, I couldn't be towed if I was there past 2 PM. All this research allowed me to build a plan.

Before school started, I went downtown to assess the parking situation. I pinpointed a few spots that would be ideal, making it easier for me to get into the building. I knew that I had to get to campus early if I had any chance of finding one of the spaces I had identified. So, every day, I would leave my home at 4:30 in the morning so that I could get downtown by 6:00 AM. Even so, I still collected many parking tickets because even the cops didn't know about the handicapped license plate regulations. At first, I was going in almost every week to contest a parking ticket, but later, I just gathered a few at a time and fought them all together.

Law school was completely different from undergraduate classes. The classrooms were much bigger, like the lecture halls at the Lincoln Park campus. There were steps to go down to the front, so I always had to sit in the back. In all my classes, I never noticed another person with a visible physical disability. I looked for racially diverse students, and I only noticed a few. The makeup of the classes was mostly white with about 60 percent of the students being male. I immediately joined the Latino Law Student Association, but it was a very small group. We met a couple of times per semester, but it was more for networking to find jobs once students were about to graduate. I couldn't relate at all.

I did make a couple of friends. It was interesting that I ended up being friends with two diverse students. One student, Tim, was white, but he was in his fifties and already had a family. He was so smart and focused. The other student, Sheila, was a beautiful black woman who was in her 30s. She joined Tim and me later during our first semester of law school. The three of us were first-year students, so we had the same classes. We had a lunch break so we would meet to go over material and eat.

The cafeteria was huge. It was on the top floor and it was used by undergraduate, graduate, and law students. I ate a lot of bagels and bananas that year, because I found out that they were the easiest to carry without risk of dropping or falling. The students at the Loop campus were different than the ones at Lincoln Park. They seemed more self-absorbed and not as social. The climate was not welcoming, so I felt very uncomfortable asking for help. I was struggling to fit in, and I was having a hard time with my confidence and comfort.

Academically, I started to see grades I had never seen. I was struggling because of my lack of access to the library. I was not able to enter the library because the elevator skipped the sixth and seventh floor where the library was located. Apparently, the elevators were designed this way to prevent law students from stealing books. The library was useful for any student, but to study law, it was imperative. I questioned the lack of access and was told that there was an elevator that would stop but an operator would have to use a key. The elevator operator was only available at certain hours and those hours conflicted with my schedule.

On some days, I was still driving Gerardo and Jaime to school when they had classes at the downtown campus. I was trying to figure out a solution, so I asked Jaime, "Would you like to make some money helping me?" He said, "What do you want me to do?" I said, "Want to kill a few trees for me?" With a puzzled face, he says, "Want me to do what?" I said, "Seriously, I need you to copy articles and cases from the law library." He said, "You don't have to pay me; I will help you." I said, "I want this to be a serious commitment so I would prefer to pay you." I ended up paying him ten dollars an hour, using the stipend money. I would give him a list of articles and cases, and he would go to the library, find the material, and make copies. Half the time, what he copied for me was useless because the material ended up not being appropriate for what I needed.

Hiring Jaime helped a bit, but it was not enough. I felt so disadvantaged not having the library available to me. My grades were reflecting my lack of case-law knowledge. Tim and Sheila tried to help; however, they were too busy doing their own work. I noticed that in law school, each student was looking out for him- or herself and no one else. It was a very competitive environment. Between paying for Jaime's time, paying for photocopies, paying for food in the cafeteria, and paying for gas money, the stipend was hardly enough.

Gerardo and Jaime continued being my good friends. We often coordinated times for us to go home together, which I appreciated because I sometimes was concerned about driving alone at night. I was highly stressed and really liked winding down from a long day with my two friends. One evening, Gerardo, Jaime, Rick, and I planned to go get pizza at Giordano's, which was next door to DePaul, before going home. The long day went fast because I had something to look forward to that evening. When we met, I said, "Ready for some pizza?" They look at each other and Jaime said, "We already ate." In an angry tone I said, "What? Are you serious?" Gerardo quickly explained, "Well, someone had a feast at a meeting on the ninth floor, and they left a lot of food in the hallway, so we served ourselves." I didn't say anything and started walking outdoors. I then said, "Thanks a lot!" Gerardo saw me notably angry and then said, "We can go eat again. Jaime and Rick, we're hungry, aren't we?" Jaime and Rick, following Gerardo's lead, nodded yes. Angrily, I said, "Forget it. I will just go to a drive-through." In unison, the three of them said, "But Giordano's doesn't have a drive-through, Pascuala." They started laughing, and though I was mad, I burst out laughing too.

Besides the stress, I was missing my family terribly. Everything that I did was related to law school. I missed family events and gatherings. My family was growing, and I couldn't celebrate with them. I was stressed all the time and was constantly out of the house. I left my house at 4:30 AM and wouldn't get home until 10 PM. My family was so supportive and tried to understand the importance of my focus. My dad wouldn't go to bed until I got home. Every day, he would be in the back room looking out the window to see when the garage light would turn on. One day, when he looked out the window, he saw the garage light on, but he also saw a tall man in a hoodie inside our yard looking into the garage. My dad immediately thought the worst and became concerned about my safety. He ran outside to make sure that I was OK. When the man saw him, he took off running out of the yard and into the alley. I saw my dad running as I came out of the garage. I didn't know what was going on. I stayed in the yard until my dad came back. He was out of breath and said, "Are you OK? Did he hurt you?" I said, "Who?" "The man who ran out of here," he responded in an agitated voice. I was concerned for my dad's well-being and said, "I'm OK. I didn't even see anyone." We both went inside.

At about midnight, a couple of hours after I'd gotten home, my mom came to my room when she saw that I still had the lights on. She said, "Something is wrong with your dad. He is having a hard time talking." I grabbed my crutches and went to my parents' room. The first thing I noticed was that my dad's mouth looked like it was drooping, which was probably why he couldn't speak clearly. I told my mom that we needed to call an ambulance because something was wrong with him. I woke Rique up and told him to go with my mother in the ambulance and that I'd follow in my car.

My dad ended up having a stroke. His left side was affected. Fortunately, he was able to go to therapy and regain some of his ability to move his arm and leg. The great shock and worry about me possibly being hurt was too much for him to handle. We noticed that our neighborhood had started to change. It didn't feel safe, and it angered me that this had happened. My dad insisted that we move because he wouldn't like it if something bad happened to us. Though we loved our home, my parents decided to look for another one. My dad worked in Franklin Park and we also knew of people from La Purísima who lived there. We sold our two-flat for $120,000, tripling what we had bought it for. With that money, we were able to purchase a small two-bedroom ranch-style home in Franklin Park. I was happy that the house only had one step to get in. It was getting difficult for me to climb the stairs all the time. The only bad thing about the move is that it added more travel time to my commute. I didn't complain, though, because all I cared about was knowing that my dad was going to be OK.

That incident changed his life. From then on, he began to slow down. Because of the stroke, he had severe neuropathy and was forced to retire. We were concerned that the change would be difficult for him, especially because he was so accustomed to traveling on the CTA bus. It took some adjustment, but after a few months, he recognized that it was a good move. He ended up loving the new home, feeling like the richest man in the world because he had never imagined having his own home all paid off.

I began to question if all the sacrifices I was making were worth it. I noticed that I was not enjoying law school. It caused me so many stresses, especially because of the Socratic method that the professors used. The Socratic method was based on asking and answering questions to stimulate critical thinking and to draw out ideas and underlying presuppositions. I dreaded being called on. I think that the professors noticed my visible fear and called on me often. Maybe they were intentionally trying to teach me that it was a cutthroat profession where one does whatever it takes to get to the top. But I realized that it was not fun to constantly be in an atmosphere that reminded me of my disability. I even started to question my interest in law. Every day I was reminded that I didn't fit the image of a lawyer in the way I looked, dressed, or even thought. I wondered if I would ever be hired, simply because I represented everything that a lawyer was not.

One assignment in my Constitutional law class really challenged me and possibly pushed me to question whether I had chosen the wrong career. The professor was covering the famous court case on abortion, Roe vs. Wade. She asked each of us to select a stance regarding our own personal view of abortion. She asked us to defend our view using existing arguments and cases. I spent the entire week preparing my pro-life argument, based on my Catholic upbringing. Jaime, who was still helping me get material from the library, probably killed a couple more trees making copies for me for this assignment. I spent several all-nighters preparing the best argument possible. As we were about to turn in the assignment, the professor said, "Hold on. The assignment isn't done yet." I looked around the class and noticed that everyone was as puzzled as I was. The professor then said, "And you thought you were done? Well, you aren't. The real assignment is to find arguments against what was written on the paper you were just about to turn in." I thought to myself, how am I supposed to do that when I wrote such a strong argument? Furthermore, it highlighted how, in law, there was no right or wrong, just what can be proven. I speculated on whether, in the long run, I would be content sometimes defending what went against my own values.

My first year was not as successful as I had hoped. Though I still didn't know my grades, I knew they were not going to be like any grades I had ever seen before. I knew that I did my absolute best, but I was so limited because of the lack of accessibility. I was glad to get a summer break away from law school. During those months, I had to decide whether to return for my second year or not. I knew that I wanted to help make the lives of people with disabilities better, but I started to entertain other possible ways that I could do that. I left campus thinking, *I want to have fun this summer, but I also need a job.* I called Mr. McGraw from DRS because, after I finished my bachelor's in sociology, he told me to contact him if I ever needed help finding a job. He referred me to an employment agency, IAM CARES, that specialized in assisting individuals with disabilities in finding jobs, and I immediately scheduled an appointment.

IAM CARES was located near the University of Illinois at Chicago. I arrived over thirty minutes early since I didn't know how the parking situation would be. I had learned how to plan and prepare for lack of access, and this preparation often resulted in me being the first one to arrive. But I guess I should have assumed that access would be more readily available since their clients were individuals with disabilities. I met with the manager, Jill. After small talk, and a few questions, Jill said, "I already looked at your resume. I got approval to hire a person to help us here in IAM CARES. Is this something that would interest you?" I asked, "What are the responsibilities for this new position?" She said, "Meeting with individuals with disabilities and supporting them with resumes, the job search process, and possibly arranging for a job coach." The first thought I had was, *why do I feel relieved?* I responded quickly and said, "Yes. I think it would be a great position for me." She then said, "You're hired."

Working at IAM CARES made me feel back at home. I felt so comfortable in my job because my disability ended up being an asset in what I was hired to do. I felt that I didn't have to worry about how I would be perceived because I was welcomed disability and all. The climate seemed so different from law school. I'd felt so out of place in law school, like I always had to prove my worth and ability. The pressure was so high that I was a nervous wreck all the time. I wasn't enjoying what I was learning, nor was I enjoying my family and friends. With this job, however, I worked my normal forty hours a week and then had evenings and weekends to enjoy life. I decided to go talk to Dr. Rafaela, my mentor at DePaul, about my situation. I needed her input to know what I should do.

I scheduled a late afternoon visit with Dr. Rafaela. I explained exactly how I was feeling. She empathized with me and said, "I agree; you should not do something that makes you so unhappy." I began to cry and shared how disappointed I was with myself for being in this situation. I said, "What will I do with a major in sociology and a minor in philosophy?" She handed me a tissue and asked, "Have you ever considered getting a master's?" I didn't have to answer before she continued, "I just read about a grant opportunity for bilingual individuals." She caught my attention immediately and I said, "Please tell me more." She continued to talk as she searched for something on her cluttered desk. "It's a master's in education in bilingual education, and all the student has to do is teach one semester as a bilingual educator in the Chicago school." My tears stopped flowing because I realized that I had a way out of law school.

Dr. Rafaela helped me complete the application paperwork and said she was sure I was going to be accepted. Though I still felt a bit disappointed, I was again feeling hope. I had always felt comfortable with both Spanish and English, so teaching one semester didn't seem too difficult. I continued working at IAM CARES for the remainder of the summer. Dr. Rafaela worked on having me accepted and registered for my new master's in education. I also notified DePaul of my decision to not return to law school and thanked them for the opportunity and the fellowship.

That summer, I spent a lot of time catching up with my family. I had nieces and nephews that were at a fun age. I would take a group, as many as could fit into my Chevy Citation, to children's museums, movies, and the zoo. One time, I took six kids, ranging in ages from eight to thirteen. My siblings trusted me with their kids and appreciated the time I spent with them. I was like a drill sergeant. As soon as they were buckled in, I would go over the rules, warning them that if the rules were broken, I would take them home and never take them again. For the most part, they were compliant.

During one of our outings, on our way back home from the zoo, my nephew, Lalo's child Orlando, was tired and not listening. He was bothering another nephew while I was driving. I told them to quit fighting. When we were about three blocks from home, in a stern voice I said, "Quit right now, or I will open the door and let you out!" Orlando responded, "So!" I had to follow through with my threat, so I pulled over, opened the door, and told him to get out. It was a scare tactic; I was just going to go around the block and then come back to pick him up. When I let him out, I went around the block as fast as I could, but when I came back around again, he was nowhere to be seen. I started to panic, going multiple times around each block. I was nervous and worried. After fifteen minutes of looking around for him, I decided to go home so that I could notify the police. As I quickly parked and told the kids to get out and rushed to go inside to call the police, I couldn't believe my eyes. Orlando was sitting in the kitchen eating cookies that my mom had given him. That little stinker taught me a big lesson, and I never did that ever again.

Certainly, I made up for lost time with my beautiful nieces and nephews. It was interesting that all of them loved me and never questioned or mentioned my disability. I know that strangers would sometimes stop in their tracks to stare, wondering if there was an "adult" with the group. Fortunately, I never cared much for people's stares, so they didn't bother me. It was also convenient because once we moved to Franklin Park, all my siblings followed us and moved close by. At one time, we had five of our families living within a couple of blocks of my mom, with three on the same street and another a block away. Jokingly, I would say, "We cannot complain about our mayor because we put him in office with the Herrera vote."

My job at IAM CARES was great. Summers always seemed to go fast, but this August arrived faster than ever. I loved working on resumes with the clients. Computers were becoming utilized more in the workplace. Jill was impressed with how fast I learned how to use the software on the mainframe computer. Each week I was given more responsibilities. I especially loved going out into the field to various work sites to observe the job coaches and clients. I'd assess whether the match was working or not. If I thought that the client wasn't connecting with their coach, I would discuss it with Jill, and she would determine if a switch was necessary. I felt knowledgeable, as if my own personal experience with my disability had prepared me more than any class I had ever taken.

The only mishap that occurred during that summer was on my way home from work. I had left the parking lot and was proceeding to Interstate 290 when I had to stop for a red light. Suddenly, quicker than I could react, a young man broke my passenger window and grabbed my purse, which I'd had on the floor. I was fortunate that there was no car in front of me because, without thinking, I accelerated forward, with the guy still hanging in my car. He fortunately got out once he had my purse in his possession. I knew that there were several housing projects near where I worked, but I had never been scared. I didn't know what to do, except to try to get out of the area. I got on the highway and headed home, but each bump would knock more glass out. I arrived home all startled, and my parents worried for me. My brother Rique went with me to the Franklin Park police station, but we were told we had to make the report where the incident took place. We did put in a report, but I knew that there wasn't much they could do; because I was so scared and things happened so fast, I wasn't able to give a description of the assailant. I reported my credit cards stolen and went to get a new driver's license. As a poor college student, I didn't have much money in my purse either.

A few weeks later, Javier, one of my DePaul friends called me. He said, "Pascuala, did you lose your purse?" I said, "Well, it was stolen." He said, "Someone called me and said that they found your purse by an elevator shaft in the projects, and he wanted me to go pick it up." I said, "Strange. Please don't go, but if he calls again, tell him to call the detective because he would go pick it up." I gave him the detective's name but, as I suspected, the person never called Javier again.

Sadly, the summer came to an end, so I had to say my goodbyes to IAM CARES. I felt sad, and I was surprised by these feelings. I feared starting my master's program and going through the same experience like in law school. I didn't want to feel like I was wasting another year by taking classes that didn't count. I didn't want to feel like my experience had been an entire waste of time. However, I was encouraged knowing that I would be back on the Lincoln Park campus and wouldn't have to collect parking tickets again or deal with an inaccessible building. As I often did, I just tried to deal with what was in front of me and didn't anticipate the future too much. I always told myself, *Just work hard and God will guide you where you need to be.* So that was exactly what I intended to do.

CHAPTER 13

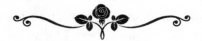

The same day I was supposed to enter my second year of law school, I started the first day of my master's program. Although the environment was familiar, it felt different. It felt like the day I first started college, full of fears, wondering if I was good enough. The year of law school had really affected my confidence and now I doubted my ability to be successful. When I told my friends from law school, Tim and Sheila, they were shocked to learn I was not going back. They'd seen how hard I'd worked and thought that it was unfair that the access was so poor. Talking to Tim helped me to calm down. He said, "Pascuala, you were a survivor and never gave up. Anyone who had to put up with not being able to use the law library would have quit on day one, but you didn't." He then told me something I will never forget: "I don't doubt that you will succeed, and whatever you do, you will make a difference."

During the first few weeks of my master's program, my stomach hurt with nerves just like it had when I'd first arrived in Chicago from Mexico. As a child, the nerves had made me throw up, but as an adult, I knew better how to control those feelings. I kept scolding myself, telling myself to stop being so silly. I couldn't help but feel this way until I took my first exams and saw that I was capable of receiving good grades just like I had in the past.

One of my favorite classes was special education. I learned about the laws that protected individuals with disabilities, and my professor shared that disabled activists were trying to pass a law to give civil rights to individuals with disabilities. This class intrigued me, so once again I went to talk to Dr. Rafaela and ask her some questions.

I went to Dr. Rafaela's office, which was always so cluttered that I was afraid of tripping on something and falling. From the doorway, I told her how much I liked the classes and that my favorite one was the special education class. She shared that DePaul offered another education major that more closely aligned with what interested me. She said, "One concentration you might like is Reading and Learning Disabilities." However, she reminded me of the specifications of the master's in bilingual education where I committed to teaching for a semester in Chicago. I asked, "Can I take more classes like the special education class?" She responded, "Yes, but the grant will not cover the cost." She saw my disappointment and continued, "Let me think and find out if there is a way you can do that master's instead."

The following week I met with her again. Dr. Rafaela looked very content, as if she had figured out a way to save me. She said, "I have an idea!" She shared information about a DePaul program, the Bridge Program, that supported students who were conditionally accepted to DePaul because of their academic background. I wasn't sure where she was headed, so I just listened intently. She said, "I was talking about you to the Director of the program and together we came up with a possible solution. The Director just received approval to hire another person for the Bridge Program because she wants to extend the program for transfer students also." Excitedly she then said, "She is willing to interview you based on my recommendation." I was still puzzled. What did this have to do with me wanting to do my master's in another concentration? She said, "If you are hired, it will be full-time, which means you can take *any* class for free. But this won't be easy, because you have to work during the day and take classes at night." I sighed but then said, "Well, I practically had fifteen-hour days at the law school, and if it's something I enjoy, I know I can do it." My interview went well, and I was hired as Associate Director of the Transfer Bridge Program.

In this position, I was responsible for assisting the Director and was charged with supporting transfer students who were admitted on a conditional basis. The students were required to take an additional class that provided supplemental support, so I became the instructor for this class that met three times a week. I worked on developing the curriculum, focusing primarily on offering study skills strategies.

The first time I taught in a classroom was intimidating. I noticed that the students didn't expect to see a Latina as their teacher, much less a Latina on crutches. But I worked hard to build trust. Students seemed resistant at first because this was a class they were required to take. However, over time, they began to get more comfortable and appreciated the support I gave them.

One day, I was teaching strategies for writing an attention-grabbing paper. I was sitting in front of the classroom but decided to stand to go write on the blackboard. I don't know how, but suddenly I slipped and fell in front of the classroom. I had to act quickly and not lose their respect. As soon as I fell, I regained composure and said, "I just got your attention, didn't I? You have to do the same on a paper." The students were not sure how to react to my comment. Still sitting on the floor, I said, "I bet no other teacher has ever demonstrated a concept like I did." This second comment gave them permission to giggle. I then said, "All kidding aside, can you please go get the security guard so he can assist me in getting up?" A couple of the male students stood up and one said, "We can help." They were strong and didn't have any difficulty pulling me up.

Just like I had done many times, I wouldn't let myself have a reaction to what had happened in class until later, when I was alone. I was angry and frustrated that I had fallen in front of everyone. I felt embarrassed and humiliated. No matter how many falls I had, I never got accustomed to the feelings that came from them. Sometimes, I felt that the emotional toll was more damaging than any physical injury. I hated that I was constantly reminded of my disability no matter how hard I worked to be just a normal, ambitious Latina woman. But that heaviness in my heart was once again pushed down and ignored. I turned my attention to a goal to accomplish. The goal now was to become the best possible instructor for this supplemental course.

Plus, now that I had this full-time job, I was able to begin my master's in reading and learning disabilities. I loved all my classes and became fascinated by so-called invisible disabilities, wondering how many people may have had a disability without my knowing. I reflected on my Spalding days, and it clicked why many of the students in my classes seemed to keep asking questions over and over. I always thought that some of their struggles were because they didn't spend time studying. Now, I more fully understood that these students likely had learning disabilities that limited their ability to process information as quickly as I did.

My days were long and exhausting. I worked full-time and took four classes. I would leave my home around 7 AM to start work at 8, and my last class ended at 9:30 PM. I would stay up studying until past midnight, and then do it all over again the next day. I used the weekends to catch up with reading and writing any papers that were due. I think I thrived when I had these types of schedules because it kept me from asking questions about my life, my fears, and my future. I just continued doing what I had learned very well—work hard, accomplish goals, and numb any scars that my disability caused, time after time. People around me never knew my real feelings but instead saw me as a strong person who wouldn't rest.

The master's degree was supposed to be a three-year program, but I wanted to finish it as soon as possible. I took classes year-round and completed the master's in two years. I loved every class and earned an A in each one. The lowest grade I received was an A-. The professor said, "Pascuala, I am going to give you an A- because when they see that you don't have an exact 4.0 GPA, they will know you worked for the grade." I'm not sure if I should've fought that, but I didn't. To manage getting As, I didn't sleep much. At times, when I knew I had to study for an exam or write a long paper, I would pack a bag with clothes and ask the custodian to lock me up in one of the classrooms.

I would study all night, taking advantage of the reduced commute time for a few additional hours to study. In the morning, I would go to the bathroom to change and wash up. My parents were concerned but, especially after my disappointment with law school, they just supported what I thought was best.

My master's program included three practicums where I utilized what I learned in my courses to evaluate a student for learning disabilities or work on remediating the issues a student with a learning disability may be having. I was also able to practice testing others for learning disabilities. I tested many of my friends and family. It was interesting to share my findings, and they felt that what I shared made sense to them.

I also practiced what I was learning in my job. Besides teaching the supplemental instruction class, I also worked with students one-to-one in supporting them. Robert, a student in the Transfer Bridge program, had transferred from a college in New York. I fully understood what learning disabilities looked like when I worked with him. He was so intelligent and articulate. He spoke with an elaborate and sophisticated vocabulary better than I would ever be able to use. However, when I looked at his writing, I would assume that an elementary school child wrote it. I couldn't believe how such an intelligent young man couldn't spell simple words. With this experience, I fully understood that a learning disability was more than just the characteristics that my textbooks outlined.

Though I had the privilege of working with Robert, not every student whom I supported had a diagnosed learning disability. I liked my job, and was making decent money, but wondered if I should consider finding a specific position that required my master's degree. Still, I was too busy to even consider the possibility of looking for a job. I was going to graduate, and then after graduating, I could sit back and think about my next step. I was looking forward to finishing my master's degree in a couple of months.

One day in May, on my way to work, I stopped at a red light at Fullerton and Ashland. Out of the blue, a young boy, about ten years old, knocked on my window. He said, "Want to buy a paper? It's only twenty-five cents." I rolled my window a bit lower and gave him a dollar, telling him to keep the change. I threw the paper on the passenger seat and kept going. Later in the day, I went to my car to have lunch. I sometimes did that just to get out of the office. I ate my sandwich and then noticed the paper, *La Raza*. I wasn't expecting it to be a fully bilingual paper. I leafed through it and then went to the job ads, just out of curiosity. One of the ads got my attention. It read: *Learning Disability Specialist, Harper College, Palatine, Illinois. Tenure Track Position.* I continued reading, and the job description was so like everything I was learning, it might as well have come straight out of my many syllabi. I had no clue where Palatine was, but I thought, *What the heck, I will send in my resume for good practice.* Later that evening, I created a cover letter and sent my resume to the address listed on the ad. I really wasn't expecting anything and forgot all about it.

I guess job hunting was on my mind after all, although I wasn't stressing about it because I had a job I was enjoying. It provided a good salary and benefits. In fact, I had just purchased a brand new red 1990 Chevy Cavalier, in my own name! I started to fantasize about possibly living on my own if a job opportunity was available in another state. I applied for a position at Notre Dame University in Indiana. When I was selected for a job interview, they scheduled me for a six-hour interview on a Friday and booked a room in one of the dorms for me to stay in overnight. I asked Gerardo if he could drive me there; part of the reason he said yes was that I'd bribed him with the fact that he'd be able to drive around in my car after he dropped me off until he picked me up the next afternoon.

My parents were not too happy with the idea of my possibly moving away and living in Indiana. My mom asked, "Alone in another state?" I replied, "I am just going to see if it is a good opportunity." In a frustrated voice she said, "Para que, hija?" I told her, "Don't worry; it doesn't mean I am taking the job for sure." My parents, as always, supported my decision, knowing that I was stubborn and had to figure things out on my own. I packed a change of clothes and went to bed.

As we had planned, I picked Gerardo up at 6 AM, thinking that would give us plenty of time to get there for an interview at 10 AM. When I saw Gerardo coming out, I slid over to the passenger side since he was going to be the driver. We took off, and he said, "Guess we're going south?" I replied, "Yes, Indiana is south." This gave me confidence that he would know how to get me there without any problems. We got on the highway, listening to Los Bukis, who continued to be my favorite. By this time, Gerardo was used to listening to Los Bukis though I never heard him sing to any of their songs. After driving south for a while, he said, "So do you have the directions?" I looked at him in disbelief, and asked, "Didn't you look up the directions since you were going to drive?" He said, "Nope, because I thought you had them." He saw my worry, and said, "Don't worry, I am sure that when we arrive in Indiana there will be a sign to Notre Dame." That comment reassured me, and I began to relax.

After a long while I said, "Have you seen the sign for Indiana?" He replied, "No, but I haven't been paying too much attention." He then said, "At the next exit I will get out to buy a map." I told him, "Good idea." We got off at the next exit, and he pumped gas while I went to the restroom. When I got out of the bathroom, he was waiting with a map in his hands. He said, "Well, Pascuala, I have some bad news, and some good news. What do you want to hear first?" I smirked and said, "The bad news." He said, "So, it looks like we're in Michigan." I said, "Oh no, I am going to be late to the interview." With a chuckle he said, "It's more like you will miss your interview." He saw my disappointed face and then said, "But here is the good news!" He asked, "Have you ever seen the movie *When Harry Met Sally?*" Not knowing how this had anything to do with what was going on, I responded, "Yes, I think so." Excitedly he says, "Well, like Harry and Sally, you and I can go to New York because that is much closer than Indiana." Without thinking, I said, "Cool! I don't know what I was thinking. I don't want to move to Indiana."

Before getting back into the car, I called Notre Dame to withdraw from the interview. We drove a bit longer and then stopped for lunch at Wendy's. I don't know if it was my hunger or my excitement, but Wendy's had never tasted so good. We drove a few hours, talking about silly and serious topics. We were so innocent in our plans. We hadn't thought about where we would stay; we hadn't considered that Gerardo had no clothes except for the ones he was wearing. The excitement of the adventure was all that mattered to us. Gerardo said, "I wish we had a camera." I asked, "Why?" He said, "Well, we need to take a picture with the Statue of Liberty." With a smile I said, "We can buy one. I have my credit card." After a couple of hours, we noticed that the map Gerardo bought was just of Michigan. I suggested that we stop and buy another map to ensure that we are going in the right direction.

This stop was like déjà vu. Again, he was looking at a map when I came out of the restroom, telling me the exact same words about good and bad news. I rolled my eyes and said, "Now what?" He said, "We are not going to New York because we are too far off. But the good news is that we can leave the country." His excitement was almost uncontrollable. We got back in the car, and again, like two little kids, we didn't think about anything other than our fun adventure. For example, no thought came to mind about not having passports or insurance when driving in another country. We kept joking around, listening to the music, and we were simply excited that we were going to Canada. When he looked at the map, he saw that we had two options. One option was to go to Niagara Falls and the other option was to go to Toronto. Before I responded, he said, "Let's go to Toronto because if we go to Niagara Falls, no one will believe we got lost." I nodded in agreement, and said, "You have a point."

It was getting dark by the time we got to the border. We showed our drivers' licenses and were able to cross into Canada very easily. We had been driving for over twelve hours, so we went to McDonald's for dinner and to stretch. Gerardo told me that the main road in Toronto was Young Street, so he wanted to make sure we got on that road.

He said, "Before we take a tour, I should call home and let them know I am not coming home for the night." I said, "I don't have to call my parents because they are not expecting me until tomorrow." We then proceed to find a phone booth. The night was chilly, so we both squeezed in together. He dialed his number, and his mother answered the call. He asks, "Mami, guess where Pascuala and I are?" She responded, "Where?" With much excitement Gerardo said, "Canada!" His mom didn't respond but rather said, "Gerardo y Pascuala estan en Canada." His father must have taken the phone and started screaming, "What the hell are you doing in Canada? And with Pascuala? You come home this instant. Do you hear me?" Gerardo, trying to calm his father down, said, "Si, Papi." He then promised his dad that we were returning home right away.

With a saddened face, Gerardo said, "We can't leave without at least going down Young Street." We drove down the street and took a fast tour, then we turned around and headed back home. Of course, we didn't count on having more difficulties crossing the US border. When we got there, they asked for passports, and like we had done before, we showed our drivers' licenses. The agent said, "This is not a valid way to show your citizenship. You need a passport or birth certificate." I started to panic and thought, *If my parents find out, they will kill me.* I worried about having to call them to fax my naturalization certificate. Gerardo, for some reason, had his birth certificate in his wallet. Perhaps he carried it because he was in the Marines. Of course, I didn't. When we told the officer that I had neither, in a loud reprimanding voice he said, "Where were you born?" Thoughts raced through my head and I worried that if I said I was born in La Purísima, I'd never be allowed to cross. Instead, I responded with the first thing that came to my mind, "I was born in the USA."

The agent was now more convinced that something fishy was going on. He began to throw out accusations and said, "You don't even speak English; where are you from?" I began to cry and couldn't respond. Gerardo talked on my behalf and said, "Of course she speaks English. She even teaches it. Pascuala, show him your paystub."

Nervously I looked in my purse and showed him that I had just been paid that same day. The agent realized that I did live in Chicago and that we were just two crazy young adults. He let us through.

As I sighed in relief, Gerardo started to scold me and said, "Don't let anyone intimidate you like that. You let that agent belittle you, erasing all your accomplishments." I began to cry, tears rolling down my cheeks. Gerardo jokingly began to sing, "I was born in the USA / I was born in the USA." I couldn't help but laugh as he sang the Bruce Springsteen song. We soon forgot about the tense experience and began enjoying our road trip again. I noticed that he was getting sleepy after driving about sixteen hours straight, so I began to develop silly games to keep him entertained. We arrived back at his home at 6 AM, exactly 24 hours from the time we'd left. I dropped him off and wished him luck with his parents. I arrived at my house thirty minutes later. My mom was up already and said, "I didn't expect you to be home until later. What happened?" Without looking up, I said, "I didn't like Indiana. I am going to get some sleep."

I smiled throughout the weekend, but I felt a little guilty also. After the fact, I thought of all that could have gone wrong. I couldn't believe that we had not considered where we would sleep. I also wondered how it went at Gerardo's home and worried that his parents would think negatively about me.

I never told anyone about this crazy adventure until many years later. But I knew that it would go down as an unforgettable experience. It was going to be one of my most memorable days ever, because I had been totally uninhibited. My disability hadn't been an issue, and for those twenty-four hours I wasn't the girl who'd had a dozen surgeries and so many broken bones. I was the girl who was living on the spur of the moment. No one could ever take that away from me.

CHAPTER 14

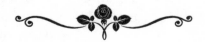

I'd totally forgotten about my application to Harper College. But one day, someone from the college called my house and left a message. When I returned the call, I scheduled a phone interview with them. I didn't think it was appropriate for Harper to call me at my current job, especially because I didn't want the Director to know I had applied elsewhere. I asked them to call me after 4 PM and gave them the number of a public telephone that was just outside one of my classrooms. I was by the phone ten minutes early, waiting for it to ring. When I spoke to them, I answered most of the questions quickly and without hesitation because they all related to the classes I was taking. I also shared my experiences with my position in the Bridge program.

Just a few days later that week, I received another message from Harper. When I called back, I scheduled an in-person interview. I set it up for the following week because I wanted a chance to drive up there beforehand since I had no idea where Palatine was. I was used to the city, and the only suburb I traveled to was Franklin Park. Rique agreed to go with me on a Saturday. It was a huge campus. We struggled to find the correct building where the interview would be held. It was a hot day, so after all the walking, I was sweating. I thought to myself, *Don't wear something too warm next week.* I also decided where to park and figured out where I might rest so that I wouldn't arrive all out of breath for the interview. I asked Rique if he knew what tenure track was, and he said he didn't. I said, "I hope it's not a job where I have to go around a track." I would certainly ask someone at work what that meant.

My interview was with the same five people that I had spoken to on the phone, and many of the questions were like what I had already been asked on the phone. I felt very comfortable and at ease with the members of my search committee. After my interview with the group, I met with Joan, the Student Development Dean. We started with small talk. She laughed when I said, "I love how the ducks just walk freely. I don't see that in the city." She said, "Oh, the geese are a nuisance around here." She asked me some questions, which I answered directly and honestly. However, I was concerned about how I responded to one question. She asked, "Why should I hire you?" I didn't even hesitate and said, "Because it's fate." I went on to tell her about the boy who sold me the newspaper that morning and how I hadn't even been looking for a job. But I hoped that she had not been turned off by my answer. I wasn't sure if they liked me, but I was glad I had interviewed. I was excited about possibly working in the field I was studying, and it excited me that I would be working on helping students with access in their classes. I knew that, since the Americans with Disabilities Act (ADA) had just been passed, colleges would be working on how to implement it.

It took a couple of weeks for Joan to call me to offer me the job. I was so excited. And, the salary was going to be ten thousand dollars more than what I was currently making. I don't know if I screamed, but it was difficult for me to contain myself. I reminded her that I wouldn't be finishing my classes until August, right before beginning in my new position. She suggested that I meet with Tom, the Director of the Center for Students with Disabilities (CSD) so that we could plan my training. I thanked her and called my mom right away. She couldn't believe that I was going to make so much. She was so happy for me because she knew how hard I had worked.

In early August, before the fall semester started, I met with Tom. Immediately, I felt comfortable. Tom's office was so peaceful, and just by observing his wall hangings, I knew he was a man of faith. That comforted me. We talked about my position and how it was a brand-new faculty position. He envisioned me having to work with faculty a lot to ensure access for students with disabilities. He explained that CSD served about 200 students and that the number of students with learning disabilities was increasing.

In August 1991, I started my full-time position as Learning Disability Specialist at Harper College. On the first day, the president of the college held a welcome meeting for the staff. New employees were introduced, and I noticed that I was one of two Latinas that started that year. I hoped that I would have an opportunity to meet Juanita, who had been hired for a position in Multicultural Affairs. I had no idea that she would become like family and someone I would love for many years. I was reassured knowing that there was a center focused on diversity. After the meeting, I had to return to my office, but since I still didn't know my way around, I decided to go to my car and drive to where my department was housed. As I was going outside, a Latino man in a suit ran to catch me. He said, "Hi, my name is Frank. Are you leaving?" I said, "I'm Pascuala, and I'm going to my office." He asked, "Can I ride with you?"

On my way to the building where CSD was, he said something that alarmed me. He said, "If you ever feel like you are not welcomed or if you are ever discriminated against, please know you can talk to me and that you have a friend." I said, "Thank you." I wanted to ask why he was telling me that, but I was afraid to find out. I did notice during the welcome meeting that there weren't many Latinos or Black people in the group. I tried not to panic, and I knew I had to work hard to prove that I was a good hire.

A faculty position doesn't come easily. I quickly learned that tenure was a privilege that had to be earned. I tried not to focus on that too much because I felt anxious each time I did. Instead, I immersed myself in my job. I quickly discovered that, at least in my center, my disability was an asset. Students seemed to connect with me quickly. They opened up to me and shared their struggles. I was empathetic and helped them to come up with solutions. But my job also required campus involvement, where I felt intimidated not only because of my disability but also because of my race.

My disability posed a challenge in other aspects of my life, although I tried to push through and not allow my mobility problems affect my participation. The campus was huge; walking from building to building became too difficult but driving to a building was too time consuming. I had to come up with a strategy that worked better for me. I decided that I would leave my manual wheelchair in my office so that I could use it to go to a meeting if it was on the opposite side of the campus. Every day, I drove my twenty-mile commute and walked in on my braces and crutches but then sat in the wheelchair only when I needed to go to a different building for a meeting.

The other faculty members in my division were counselors, and one of them, Shari, was in CSD. She was very welcoming with her quiet personality. She had an open-door approach and encouraged me to ask questions about anything. It did not take long for me to utilize her expertise as I got acclimated to my new role at the college. All the counselors were very welcoming, though I did feel out of place the first time we were on a retreat. Joan liked to gather all her employees at an off-campus location for some team building and division-planning activities. Probably within the first couple of months of starting at Harper, we had an overnight retreat for everyone in our division. I vividly remember that access had not been considered for this retreat (but after I joined the team, that began to change). The retreat center was a two-floor building, and the dining room, where meals were scheduled, was on the second level. Food had to be brought down to me, but several people chose to join me downstairs so I wouldn't be alone.

Some of the activities planned were not accessible for an individual with a physical disability like me. Don't ask me why, but we were broken into teams, and we had to go on a scavenger hunt to look for different items on a list, one of which was a buffalo. Each team had the task of locating the items and then taking a picture. This required each team to go into the surrounding area of the retreat house in a vehicle. Anita, one of the counselors, volunteered her minivan for our team to go on the hunt. I immediately recognized that I wouldn't be able to climb up into the van. Trying to please and not be a sour puss, I didn't make an issue of it. Instead, I suggested that I could sit on the floor in the back. I will admit that at times, I thought that had been a bad idea, especially when half of my butt was hanging out since we had to leave the back door open to readily be able to take a picture. Still, I was a good sport and participated as a good team member. Deep down, though, I hated having so much difficulty with the simplest of activities. Of course, no one ever figured that it bothered me because I had learned to push forward no matter what and to ignore how frustrating it was to have my disability always impacting my life.

Anita and I became friends after that team building activity. She is this spunky, full-of-life white lady who loves everything and everyone who is different. Immediately, I felt so comfortable with her, as if my race, my past, my disability, and everything else I tried to hide were not important to her. She was so open to me that I participated in some of her student programs, and she was always willing to help me find solutions for me to participate fully. She was the lead of an off-campus student retreat for which I volunteered to help. Because the Harper vehicle was not accessible, Anita and I rode separately with some students, not knowing that the trip would be the scariest ride of my life. Heading back after a successful retreat, we were caught in the middle of a blizzard where visibility was close to nothing. She was brave and kept forging through while I kept thinking to myself, *Dear God, this is not how I want to die*. After this experience, I knew that our friendship would be indestructible.

Similarly, I met a young, super fun counselor, Stephanie. Though she was younger than me, she exuded confidence, something I sometimes lacked. Like with Anita, my disability didn't affect Stephanie. They both gave me confidence because they valued my knowledge and comments. Soon after starting to work at Harper, the three of us were very invested in knowing as much as we could about diversity. We attended seminars and trainings to learn more. One trip was to Western Illinois University. I still laugh when I remember how we were not expecting to be out in the boonies. We stayed in the only motel in Macomb, Illinois. They considered Walmart to be their mall. One night, we busted out laughing when I called to report the bothersome noise outside our room. I called and said, "Is there anything that can be done about the frogs outside our room? They are not letting us sleep." With a Southern accent the man on the other end responded, "You mean the toads? No, there isn't. You can wear earplugs." We had a lot of fun. Instead of feeling like I was a nuisance when there was lack of access, they appreciated their own privilege as able-bodied women helping me to find solutions.

I worked hard, and I loved my job! Tom was such an excellent boss that he allowed me to develop and try new ideas. Just two years after I started, we began the Program for Achieving Student Success (PASS), a fee-for-service tutoring program to support our students with one-to-one tutoring. I came up with the program's name by asking a student, "If we had a program that described the support, I've given you, what would you want it to be." Quickly he said, "The PAS program. PAS for Pascuala." I smiled and thanked him. From his remark, I came up with the name. PASS was very successful, and families were willing to pay an additional fee for support for their students. I managed the program while having my own caseload of students.

I started to develop wonderful relationships with students. The ones who attended regularly loved when we would come up with strategies that helped them academically. Once, a student with memory issues was taking a botany class and was having a difficult time recalling the names of various types of leaves. I suggested he create flash cards, not only with the name of the type of leaf but also with a picture of the leaf. He took it one step further. The next time I saw him, he had laminated the actual leaf with the name spelled out on it. Another student couldn't remember how to spell numbers and was constantly making mistakes when writing checks. Together we created a wallet card outlining all the numbers and spellings, like the little cards that existed for figuring out tips.

Another student, Becky, required CSD to come up with creative solutions. She had recently been injured in an automobile accident that caused her to be quadriplegic because of her spinal cord injury. She was very artistic and wanted to pursue a degree in Fashion Design. With the limited use of her arms, we had to come up with solutions and reasonable accommodations. Fortunately, the Fashion Department faculty were willing to collaborate with us on this because they recognized Becky's tremendous talent. She successfully completed the degree and went on to get more education. It was great to see Becky's success over the years. For this reason, I nominated her as a distinguished alumna many years later. In addition, I helped to bring her project, Tres Fridas, to Harper; she and two of her friends recreated iconic pieces of art by putting individuals with disabilities as the subjects. It was great seeing how she became so successful after Harper. It was a success story that proved that sometimes the impossible can be made possible.

Sometimes my ideas to help students were not always understood or well received. Right after receiving tenure after three glowing evaluations, I was involved in a very uncomfortable situation. I was working with a student with severe dyslexia. He was in a developmental English class and was struggling to write his papers, not because he didn't have ideas, but because he would forget his idea by the time he got a word on paper and remembered how to spell it. He was very intelligent but writing and reading were so difficult because of his learning disability. Seeing all his difficulties I suggested we try something else. I said, "Pretend I'm your secretary; dictate what you want to say." As he dictated, I typed. He ended up with a great paper full of ideas. His English teacher became concerned, though, because the writing he did in the classroom was so different from what he was turning in after being helped by me. Instead of the faculty member calling me to get an explanation, she contacted her dean, who in turn contacted Tom. The dean of that department demanded a meeting to discuss the situation. Tom thought it was important for me to attend, although the issue was never communicated to me.

When we were around the table at the meeting, the dean started the conversation, and not in an amicable way. With accusation in her voice, she said, "Pascuala, we didn't hire you to cheat for your students!" I don't know where I got the confidence to defend myself, but I responded, "First, *you* didn't hire me. Harper hired me. Second, I resent you questioning my integrity when you don't even know me. You can question my methods any day, but never my integrity." I think I left her speechless because I saw her sink into her chair. She then softened her tone and said, "OK, tell us what you have been doing and why the student's papers look so different when he does them with you." I was prepared and showed her how, under the law, dictation was considered a reasonable accommodation. After discussing my method with them, I addressed the faculty member who had remained quiet. I said, "Are you more interested in spelling or in the ideas the students have?" I continued, before allowing her to answer, "Do you mark the students down for spelling?" She admitted that the development of the idea was the outcome she was after. The meeting ended with their understanding of how dictation was a reasonable accommodation.

I always saw possibilities, not impossibilities, and didn't fear thinking outside the box to help my students. I began to form my own philosophy about life and purpose. I had a bunch of ideas in my head, but a conversation with my dad clarified them for me. One day when I arrived home from work, my dad was sitting out in the yard. I said, "Hi dad, what are you doing?" While pointing to the ground, in a quiet tone he said, "Watching those ants." I waited for him to continue as I looked down at the ants he was pointing to. He said, "They are busy coming and going." I asked, "And why do you think they are busy?" He looked at me and said, "Everything that God created has a purpose. Sometimes we may not understand it, but they are on this earth for a reason." I said, "Hmmm, I never even noticed the ants." He said, "Don't forget that anything with life is valuable and should be protected." He got up, grabbed my book bag, and led me inside the house.

I have kept this conversation in my mind ever since. I held this philosophy in my work at Harper from the beginning. I thought of each student, regardless of their disability, as valuable and filled with potential. It was my job to help them figure out their purpose. Interestingly, I guess I was so busy figuring each students' purpose that I forgot to contemplate and analyze my own. As a result of this philosophy, though, I developed a reputation of always being able to help the most at-risk students. I always tried to do it with compassion, and I celebrated with them as they completed their goals.

My job at Harper came to me naturally. I felt content and well acclimated to my new environment. I was busy learning the job my first years, but afterward, I started to wonder if this was it. I felt that I needed more than just a career to fulfill me as a person and knew deep down that I was not entirely content. During the evenings, I would spend time with my growing number of nieces and nephews. There were well over a dozen young kids that looked up to me, and the outings with my munchkins continued. My sister Reyna even selected me to be the godmother of her two children, Erika and Richie. And then, my niece Vanessa, Angelita's daughter, asked me to be her godmother during her first communion.

My sister Tere lived across the street from my mom's house, so I spent a lot of time with her girls, Velia and Estela. I'm so grateful that my brother-in-law, Ismael, never hesitated in letting my nieces be with me. He even allowed them to travel as my companions, helpers, and best friends. Velia and I vacationed to Los Angeles, staying at a cousin's house who took us to Tijuana, Mexico. Another summer, Estela and I traveled to Durango, Mexico, the city and state in Mexico where I had been first diagnosed with polio.

My salary was good for someone who was single and still living at home. Though I was helping with my living expenses, I felt that I should be on my own. When I suggested that I move out, my parents resisted. They said, "This house is yours. If you are not comfortable, let us know and we can change it." I said, "I would like to have my own space and my own kitchen so that I could learn to be more self-sufficient." My dad responded, "Do whatever you want to this house." I don't know why they didn't want me to move out, but I think they worried that I wouldn't have anyone to pick me up if I fell when living on my own. I took their word and hired my cousin to remodel an addition so that I could have my own space and at least feel like I was living on my own. Of course, the whole time I was there, I think I used that kitchen only a handful of times.

Though I had a wonderful job and a great family, I couldn't help but feel an emptiness in my heart. I was not at peace and yearned for something to make me happy. I didn't admit to myself that I wanted a romantic relationship. I also continued wanting to have a greater impact on society by making the lives of people with disabilities better. Although I was making a difference in the lives of students I worked with in my office, I felt that I was not doing enough. I started to talk to people within my circle of contacts to find out if I could be involved in any social movement. I found out about a group called Disabled Americans Rally for Equality (DARE) and decided to attend a meeting just to get more information.

The DARE meeting was on the south side of Chicago, far from where I lived. The gathering was at the DARE President's home. I was shocked to find out that Doug, who was in a wheelchair and was deaf and blind, was the president. His wife was the interpreter, signing everything into his hands. At work, we had a large deaf community, so I was familiar with American Sign Language (ASL), but this was my first time meeting someone who had three disabilities. Doug was able to speak for himself since he had not lost his hearing and vision until later in life as a result of a condition called Usher Syndrome. At this meeting, they were planning on an upcoming "action," which was going to be held in San Francisco. Doug said, "We will travel from Chicago to San Francisco for a demonstration demanding rights for people with disabilities." He explained that the work was not over, even if the ADA had been signed. He explained that the funding had been secured to cover airfare, ground transportation, and hotel, in addition to a daily stipend for food. Doug asked to be notified if we were planning to go to San Francisco. He also said, "Let's see how many of us get arrested this time."

Hearing the word "arrested" scared me, though I had heard that the national organization had lawyers to get us out and that it wouldn't go on our records. I thought to myself, *Oh, I can't get arrested. I am a faculty member.* I also had to discuss it with Tom to see if I could go since it was taking place during the week. After Tom approved, I decided to go, just to check it out. I was not prepared for this experience. Traveling with at least twenty passengers that required assistance to board the airplane was chaotic at best. And, when we arrived in San Francisco, the airport was inundated with people in all types of mobility devices. I had no idea that so many people with disabilities would be participating. Special transportation had been arranged to take us to the hotel. The process of checking in was long and tedious. Imagine a small lobby with two elevators packed with at least one hundred and fifty wheelchair users. I wasn't sure if I had made the right decision to attend the trip. Many of the individuals were frequent flyers who modeled their various types of activist t-shirts. Some displayed stickers on their wheelchairs and were proud of their new paraphernalia.

During the next two days, I decided to stick close to the DARE group and follow along. I had no idea that this would mean watching how some people would get arrested and sometimes even dragged out of the way. There was nonstop chanting, and the cops on scene were unsure of how to handle some situations. I saw a young girl, Kelly, in her early twenties with severe disabilities, possibly cerebral palsy, who visibly wanted to get arrested. Her thin body appeared to be twisted and stiff, and she was not able to clearly communicate. But when I saw that Kelly was not afraid of getting arrested, I felt like a hypocrite. I asked myself, *Why am I here? If this is such an important issue, then why am I so afraid to be arrested?* At that instant, I decided to be in it fully without concern about arrests.

It felt awesome to be able to let out all my bottled-up anger. Over five hundred people of all ages from across the nation were gathered in front of a hotel where lawmakers were making decisions that affected individuals with disabilities. I was angry! I hated the limitations that had been imposed on me simply because of my disability. I demanded change and wanted it now! I chanted, "Together, United We'll Never be Defeated! Together, United We'll Never be Defeated!" I lost all fear and inhibition screaming with all my might. We teased the police as they tried to push people in power wheelchairs after they had turned off their power. We screamed, "Our disability is not contagious!" I noticed how the police officers had plastic ties instead of handcuffs to arrest people. I am certain that they were expecting us because they had special lift-equipped buses for transporting arrestees. I was transported on one of these vehicles to Pier 39 where they had temporary jail cells. I laughed as some people chanted, "We don't even have the right to be arrested." What a powerful day! I was all hyped up and I wanted more. After a successful day of over one hundred arrests, we gathered in a ballroom at the hotel to celebrate. We listened to each other's war stories and laughed at how we had disrupted the convention.

From then on, I continued attending meetings and took any action I could. At the same time, I also sought ways to meet other young adults. Shirley, my college friend, invited me to group Bible study. During one of the evening meetings, a woman, Pat, passed around information about an upcoming Life Search weekend retreat for young adults sponsored by Life Directions. Pat had previously attended and highly recommended the experience. I asked Pat for more information and decided to sign up for the retreat.

Life Directions inspires people to motivate and lead their peers to take charge of their lives. I loved their mission and hoped that I would enjoy the experience. I was concerned about access, but I hoped that the leaders of the retreat would work with me. The retreat was held in an old religious convent in Glenview, Illinois. We began with a welcome by the retreat leaders, Father John and Sister Rosalie. I was impressed with both Father John's and Sister Rosalie's pep and high energy. They worked in unison and helped each other throughout the weekend. It was interesting how these very different individuals had formed such a beneficial program. Sister Rosalie was Latina and spoke both Spanish and English fluently. I immediately noticed how she connected with every single person at the retreat. Father John was a white priest who impressed me with his energy and downright happiness. He also spoke Spanish, though not as fluently. They had cofounded the organization and told us about the different aspects of all they did. The weekend retreat was packed with activities that included prayer, music, singing, and team building. One team-building exercise posed a tremendous challenge for me.

We were paired off and directed to go out to the grounds and take turns allowing our partner to lead us while blindfolded. I was petrified of falling but insisted on participating. This activity helped me realize how privileged I was to be able to see. I also discovered that I am very trusting and that in my heart I want to believe in the goodness of people. I was pleasantly surprised when we finished this tense activity without falling. However, ironically, I fell when we were heading to dinner. I normally didn't cry when I fell, but for some reason, I felt safe to cry that time. After a couple of guys picked me up, I had to wipe the tears from my face but didn't say a word. Later that evening, I talked to Father John and again broke down and began to cry. I said, "Why is life so difficult?" I think Father John was surprised with my question but appreciated my honesty. I didn't know it at the time, but Father John and Sister Rosalie would remain in my life forever.

Life Directions became a good way for me to fill the emptiness and loneliness I felt because of how my disability made me feel. Father John recognized my leadership skills and empowered me to stop focusing on myself by instead putting my attention on others. He also became my spiritual director, meeting with me weekly. Father John challenged and pushed me to look at my life differently. Likewise, Sister Rosalie pushed me to lead and facilitate what they called life circles. Every other week, we would form a circle of young adults to read scripture and discuss how we felt about it. I became involved with this great organization when I needed it most. I was helping the students I worked with at Harper to find their purpose, but I was lost without knowing where my own life was headed.

Life was a valley of tears according to my mother, but I wasn't convinced that I had to accept that notion. I kept searching for the happiness I felt I lacked. I kept getting involved with more and more responsibilities because it prevented me from asking the questions that were so troublesome for me. My parents were so proud of me and satisfied with all my accomplishments. My brothers and sisters were also pleased with my level of education, especially because none of them had attended college. I am sure that when each member of my family recalled how polio had paralyzed me for months, and when they remembered how I had crawled around on the ground, they felt grateful for all that I had accomplished. I, too, recognized how far I had come, but asked myself, *Am I wrong for wanting more?*

I went through a period that I described as falling in love with love. I would entertain fantasies of forming a relationship with any man I encountered. Amazingly, I saw every male as a potential life partner. Literally, I befriended any person who talked to me. Seriously, anyone. For example, I even became friends with a man who dialed the wrong number and reached me instead. He called, and said, "Hi, Alicia, how are you?" I said, "I am not Alicia, but I am fine, how are you?" He responded, "I am fine. My name is Pepe." I said, "Hi Pepe, my name is Cuali." We continued conversing and asked if he could call again. I accepted. I guess that's what we had to do then instead of having cyber-relationships.

Though I easily made friends, these relationships always led to disappointment after disappointment. I even dated a guy I met at a restaurant when some of my friends and I went to dinner. His name was Tomas, and he didn't speak English. My friends thought he was acting strange, but I shushed them and told them to be nice. Tomas indeed was strange and not a good person. He used me, and when he realized I had money, he asked me to buy things for him, promising to pay me back. For instance, in Spanish he said, "I am trying to learn English. Can you buy me a VHS player so I can play some tapes for me to learn?" To please him, I did. It was not a give and take relationship. It all came crashing down when his girlfriend, yes, *his girlfriend* called me. In an angry tone she said, "Leave Tomas alone, you crazy invalid." I was in shock, totally speechless. As if that wasn't enough, she then said, "I cannot believe you bought him all those things. At night we sat and laughed, talking about how stupid you were."

I was devastated and so hurt. I thought, *I was wrong to think that I was worthy of being loved.* Before I had the chance to change my number, he called again, not knowing what had happened. I gave him a few choice words and then changed my phone number immediately. I didn't tell anyone what had happened. I just secluded myself in the biggest pity party ever; this time, no one was invited. I was in this state for a couple of weeks. I kept replaying the conversation over and over. My only diversions were work, Life Directions, and my involvement with civil disobedience.

DARE had another action planned in Washington, DC. I had been to Washington, DC, once before and I had loved it. I was certain I wanted to go. Because it was during school, no one in my family was able to accompany me. At Harper, I had developed a beautiful connection with Juanita, the other Latina who started working there when I did. Though we worked in different departments, I would always help during any Latino event. We had the same way of thinking and were both in sync with what we knew our families needed. We had lunch regularly and when I told her about my involvement with DARE, she volunteered to accompany me. I knew from then on that Juanita and I would be like sisters.

During this trip, I revisited many of the monuments and important governmental buildings like the Capitol and the White House. We protested as we always did. It was very emotional for me to participate by scooting up the steps of the Capitol. This same activist group had participated in the famous "Capital Crawl" that is said to have convinced President George H. W. Bush to sign the ADA in 1990. It brought memories of all the barriers I had faced in my life and reinforced why rights for people with disabilities were so important. Juanita's perspective was changed by all the protesting and especially by witnessing my own lack of accessibility.

CHAPTER 15

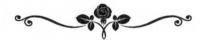

After a few disappointing relationships, I committed myself to working hard at Harper, being active with Life Directions, and continuing my involvement with DARE. I even started to take leadership roles in both Life Directions and DARE. In Life Directions, I cofacilitated the Life Search weekend retreats with Father John. For DARE, I became one of Doug's assistants. I learned how to finger spell, so I would spell out words into his hands to let him know what was happening. This gave his wife a break from having to travel with him.

During each flight, I would sit next to Doug and describe the surroundings and inform him of any announcements. I will never forget a conversation I had with him on the flight to Las Vegas. He said, "Pascuala, do you know that, with my disability, it is like living in a closet?" I asked, "How?" He responded in a serious tone, "It's like living in a closet where only one person at a time can enter and not every person can enter." I didn't interrupt and had him continue. He then said, "I live in a soundless dark closet where only one person who can sign or finger spell can enter." I appreciated his analogy because it provided me with a deeper appreciation for all that I could do and realized that, although my life had been difficult at times, I was so fortunate in so many ways. Perhaps for Doug, life had more valleys of tears than my own.

Las Vegas was a city I'd always wanted to visit. Besides participating in the social justice activities, I was hoping to try my luck with some of the slots. It excited me that the plan was to block the strip and interrupt gamblers from playing until our demands for equality were heard. Again, there were hundreds of people in wheelchairs along with personal care assistants and allies. It was early October, so the weather was a bit chilly. I wore my bright colored windbreaker and had a blanket in my backpack in case I needed it. For this trip, my sister Tere's daughter Velia had traveled with me. Because I used a manual chair, she would help to push, especially inside hotels when plush carpets made it very difficult for me. We were instructed to go as far out on the streets as possible and block the two main streets on the strip. We moved quickly and then chained ourselves together so that police officers wouldn't be able to easily move us. The usual chant began, "Together united, we'll never be defeated." We grabbed signs and continued our chanting. Some of the leaders used a bullhorn to incite us into a roar.

During a lull, a young Latino man cleared his throat and said to me, "Are you going to get arrested?" I smiled and said, "No. I want to gamble." He smiled in return and then said, "Would you mind if I gambled with you?" I thought to myself, *Wow, these are original pickup lines.* I was afraid he had read my mind, so I quickly said, "No, I don't mind." We began to chant again. I noticed that he had his legs covered with a blanket, so I wondered what his disability was. At another quiet time he said, "My name is Isidro Herrera. What is your name?" I said, "Get out of here, you must be lying!" I just couldn't believe that we had the same last name. He chuckled and responded, "No, I'm serious." I half-jokingly said, "Show me your ID," to which he obliged and took out his driver's license. I quickly saw that he was telling me the truth. Furthermore, I saw that he lived in Austin, Texas. We continued chatting, though I couldn't help but notice that he was obviously shy. I almost heard his mind turning with every word he spoke.

We were all happy with the results of our protest. We received a lot of media attention and were able to voice our demands for equality. That evening everyone was invited for a meeting and celebration. Velia and I attended but had planned to go to the casino afterward. It was interesting how Isidro had been in other cities with his group from Austin, but our paths had never crossed before. We both had been in San Francisco and Washington but had never met. He belonged to ADAPT, an activist group that started it all. For the first time, disability was being viewed as a civil rights issue. At Harper, I was working with others on diversity programming for students and for the first time, "disability" was being considered under the diversity umbrella.

Isidro followed me to the casino, and he watched me play. I'm not going to lie—I was uncomfortable at first because he didn't play, but rather, he just stared. He wasn't much of a conversationalist either. He kept clearing his throat as if to remind me that he was still there. I played the penny slots, so my twenty dollars lasted a long while. He didn't move and just watched attentively. I was tired so I said to Velia, "Let's go to our room. I'm exhausted." I wasn't sure what to say to Isidro. I didn't want to be rude and just say goodbye, so I said, "Will I see you tomorrow?" He took those words as an invitation, and said, "Yes, it's a date." Strange, but when he said that, I felt butterflies in my tummy and felt my cheeks warm.

The next day, Isidro and I saw each other while out protesting. He had a t-shirt on and began shivering because it was colder than the day before. I said, "I just bought this sweatshirt as a souvenir, do you want to borrow it since it's long-sleeved and warm?" It was a bright red sweatshirt with aces on the front. He accepted my offer and put it on. We continued talking throughout the day. He told me about Austin, where he had his own apartment. He said he worked for JCPenney doing customer service. His eyes opened wide when I shared that I was a faculty member at a community college. We talked about our respective families. We simply connected, and it felt safe talking to him. We even hung out after the protest. He was friends with his two travel mates, Wayne and Roy, who were in power wheelchairs and were clearly wilder than Isidro. I wondered if Isidro was hiding how he truly was.

For some reason, I felt sad the next day, knowing that we'd be heading to the airport to fly back to Chicago. He came out to see me leave. As the minivan was loading, we exchanged phone numbers. I got on the minivan using the lift. I looked out the window as I was being strapped and noticed him like a statue, not moving an inch. This sensation of not wanting to say goodbye came over me. I didn't understand why I was feeling like this. As the minivan took off, I kept looking out the window until I lost sight of him. Deep down, I wasn't sure if I'd see him again and that saddened me.

When I got home, I unpacked but still couldn't get him off my mind. I pulled out the card where he had written his phone number. In 1994, cell phones weren't still readily available and long-distance calls were expensive. Still, I decided to try the number he had scribbled. I called, and there was no answer until a computerized voice picked up. I hung up quickly and didn't leave a message. I tried another time a bit later and the same thing happened. I went to bed wondering if he had given me the wrong number.

The next day, I got up and got ready for church. I went to St. Gertrude Parish in Franklin Park with my parents. This church was full of people from La Purísima. Inevitably, I would hear remarks from someone commenting on the "miracle" that I was. The conversation with my mom would go something like this: "And she drives? I can't believe it," with my mom responding, "Yes, and she works at a college." The person continued with patronizing comments as if I weren't present. I learned to block out how these comments made me feel. I excused them because they probably didn't know better.

During the evening, I felt restless, going back and forth on whether I should try to call Isidro again. I turned on the television to the only semi-good program, *Siempre en Domingo*, a variety show that displayed the popular Mexican musical groups. I was antsy and couldn't focus on anything except wondering what I should do. I finally gave in and decided to dial his number. Again, the phone rang four times until the answering machine picked up. I wished that the machine would have played the sound of his voice so at least I would know if I was dialing the right number. I quickly hung up after the computerized voice picked up. I waited a couple of hours, and right before I went to bed, I decided to call one more time. This time, I had decided to leave a voice message if there was no answer. The phone rang, the machine answered, and I left the following message, "I'm trying to reach Isidro, um, if I have the right number, um, call me at this number." I left my phone number and hung up. It took me a while to fall asleep wondering why I was so insistent on reaching him.

Monday was busy, and then it was over in the blink of an eye. I was always able to focus on the students and forget anything else on my mind. When I got home, I checked to see if there was mail, had a brief conversation with my parents, and went to the back. The newly constructed mini apartment included a bedroom, a full kitchen, and a bathroom. It was a compromise my parents preferred instead of my moving out. I decorated the space to my liking. I glanced over to my phone which had a built-in answering machine and noticed there were two messages. My heart began to beat a little faster as I thought it might be Isidro. And, it *was* him. He had not given me the wrong number but explained that from Las Vegas, his group had to drive all the way back to Austin, so he was still on the road when I had tried to reach him. He said he would try reaching me the next day because he was going over to his friend's house to watch the Cowboys on *Monday Night Football*. I felt disappointed but at the same time relieved. I'd have to wait a bit longer to talk to him again.

As promised, Isidro called me again on Tuesday, but this time, I was there to pick up. We talked about our respective trips home, football, my favorite music, and anything that came to our minds. I forgot that we were on a long-distance call and didn't consider how expensive the call would be for him. After an hour, he also noticed and said that he should probably go. Before he hung up, he asked if we could talk again soon. I told him it was my turn to call, and we decided I'd call on Thursday. I went to bed and smiled about the nice conversation I had with him. I felt that he was different than any other person I knew. It felt right. I slept peacefully for the entire night.

On my way home on Wednesday, I was feeling disappointed that I wouldn't talk to Isidro until the next day. I thought about ways to get my mind off him. I arrived home and sat down to watch the novela my mom was watching. I always enjoyed las novelas and all their drama, but I disliked how all the women in them were pretty with perfect bodies. I never saw a short, chubby, disabled woman like me. I was twenty-nine and thought I would never get married, so when I watched las novelas, I often felt sad because the actresses didn't represent me in any way. As I watched that night, I heard my phone ringing in the back room. I got up as quickly as I could but missed answering the call. I watched the phone for a minute hoping a message would be left. I was going to head back to the living room with my parents when the phone rang again, and it was Isidro.

Our long-distance phone calls continued for a couple of weeks. Then, we decided to start writing to each other since we were worried about our high phone bills. No matter how often we promised not to talk every day, we ended up breaking the rule. During one conversation, I told him that one of my favorite music artists, Juan Gabriel, was going to be coming to Chicago to perform at the United Center for Thanksgiving weekend. He said, "And are you going?" I responded, "I need to find someone who will go with me." He then said, "Why don't you ask me?" I chuckled and said, "Because you're in Austin." He replied, "But there are planes." I didn't know if he was joking, but I asked, "Want to go to the Juan Gabriel concert with me?" I held my breath and couldn't believe it when he said yes.

Isidro arrived in Chicago for the long Thanksgiving break in 1994. He booked a hotel near me, which wasn't difficult since I lived by O'Hare airport. I agreed to pick him up on Wednesday night. I was so nervous! I knew part of my nerves was figuring out how to navigate the airport. I was concerned that there would be no way for me to walk the long distances, so I decided to take my wheelchair. Although it was a light wheelchair, I still struggled to get it out of the trunk. I met him by the luggage claim. When we saw each other, it was awkward because neither of us knew how to greet each other. We just smiled and said hello, and then I had him follow me to my car. When we'd first met, he was in a wheelchair, so I didn't expect him to be on crutches. His crutches were very different from mine because the bottom of them was a round circular shape.

During the weekend he wanted to meet all my family. I thought that the best way to do that would be to visit each of my siblings individually at their homes. He was very polite with each of my brothers and sisters. His Spanish wasn't fluent, but he spoke it well enough for my parents to be able to speak to him. My family was a bit confused about why I was introducing him to everyone when I had just met him the month before myself. I, too, was confused about why I would go to all that effort for someone who was supposedly just my friend. I had friends that I had known for much longer and I'd never introduced *them* to my parents or to my siblings. Why was this different?

The Juan Gabriel concert was a lot of fun for me, though I wasn't too sure it was fun for Isidro. Mexican concerts tend to be very loud with all the fans singing along. I sang, danced in my seat, and took pictures, but when I looked over at him, he was sitting still, almost like a statue. I wondered if he wasn't enjoying the show. I said, "Do you like the concert?" He said yes. I sang along to any song Juan Gabriel sang and hoped that Isidro would loosen up, but he didn't. On the way home, I asked if he liked the music and he admitted that he had never heard Juan Gabriel's music before. I realized that although he had the skin color like mine, his upbringing had been very different.

His upbringing was not the only difference between us. During those months we spent talking on the phone, I learned a lot about him. The onset of his disability happened when he was a teenager.

He was diagnosed with juvenile rheumatoid arthritis. The disability had been very painful, and it had caused him to lose the movement of his joints. He had to be in rehab to learn how to be independent again because he only had a certain range of motion. He joked that he was glad that at least he could bend one of his arms so that he could eat. The more I learned about what he had to endure, the more I admired him, because he made it sound like it hadn't been a big deal. I knew that his perspective on disability was likely different than mine. Having a disability was all I knew, but I wondered how it was for him to once be able to do something and then not to be able to do the same. I knew that he probably suffered not only from the pain his arthritis caused but also by what he suffered emotionally by having to adjust to his new limitations.

The long weekend was a whirlwind, and I felt sadness when he had to leave and go back home. I wasn't sure if or when I would get to see him again. I convinced myself that at least I had found a good friend who seemed to understand me better than anyone ever had. We promised to continue talking on the phone but to be smart about how many calls we made. Our previous month's bill had been expensive, so I understood we had to put some limitations on ourselves.

As I continued getting to know him, I was amazed by how our mutual disabilities complemented each other. He was not able to bend his joints while I was able to kiss my toes if I wanted to. He was strong and could lift heavy items while I was a weakling that barely could carry my own weight. Even with our disabilities being different, we also shared a lot of similarities. Both of us loved our families and especially our moms. In addition, we shared a strong belief in God and the power He had over our lives. Although he was not a practicing Catholic, he had all his sacraments and at one time had been a churchgoer.

During one of our conversations in December, we talked about Christmas gifts and what we were planning to do for the holidays. I told Isidro how important Christmas was for my family and how my mom had always requested Christmas to be her holiday where we would all gather at her home to celebrate. He also valued Christmas and said it was his favorite holiday. He then said, "You know what I want for Christmas?" I said, "No, what?" He took a breath and then said, "I'd want you to come to Austin." I stayed quiet, trying to assess if he was serious or not. He broke the silence and said, "Why don't you come right after Christmas and spend the New Year's holiday in Austin?" I tried to make a joke and said, "New Year's in 80-degree temperatures?" He said, "Or hotter." I didn't give him an answer that night, but the next time we talked, I told him I had his Christmas gift ready, because I was going to spend New Year's with him in Austin.

It was a bit difficult to convince my parents to let me go to Austin. Even at my age, I still asked for permission because it was part of our culture and I lived under their roof. I think they figured that I was certainly old enough to know what I was doing, so they couldn't stop me. Plus, I think it helped that they had liked Isidro when they met him and, though they never told me directly, they were glad that I had met someone like him.

I booked a hotel near where he lived in Austin. And just like he'd met my whole family in Chicago, the bulk of the time I was in Austin, I spent making the rounds to meet his parents, his four younger sisters, and his friends. We were invited to a New Year's party with his friends, Roy and Wayne, whom I had already met in Las Vegas. The party was nothing like any of the parties I had ever been to before. There was a lot of alcohol, and the music was loud. I found it amusing that Roy, who was unable to use his arms, used a straw to drink his beer.

When the party was over, Isidro took me to my hotel and asked if he could come in. I told him I had nothing to offer him in terms of drinks, but that he could come in. He sat on the edge of the bed and as he looked at me, he said, "I have a question for you." I said, "You do? What?" He grabbed my hand and said, "Will you marry me?" I burst out laughing. I said, "Stop joking around like that. We just met." He just kept quiet. I then said, "It's getting late and I think you might have drunk too many beers." He slowly got up from the bed and walked to the door. He said, "OK, good night. I will pick you up at 10 AM to take you to the airport."

The ride to the airport felt tense. It was not the same comfortable feeling I'd always experienced with him since we first met. I wasn't sure what it was, so I just remained quiet, waiting to see if he'd say something. He dropped me off at the airport, and I flew back home. I was puzzled because I didn't know exactly what went wrong. I didn't like how I felt, so I decided to call him with the excuse of letting him know I got home safely. After he picked up the phone, I said, "Hi, I just wanted to tell you that I got home." He said, "Good. I hope you had a nice flight." I responded, "Yes, I did." Then there was dead silence. It seemed long, so I finally said, "Hey, are you mad?" He coughed, and then said, "Why would I be? Because you laughed at the idea of marrying me?" I said, "What? Were you serious?" He said, "Of course I was. I'd never joke about something like that. You didn't even let me tell you that I'd give you the ring later." I couldn't believe my ears. I got proposed to. He wanted me to be his wife. I don't know why, but the only thing that came out of my mouth was, "Of course I will marry you." It scared me to think I loved him already. Was it that? Or perhaps I thought it was cheaper to get married than to keep paying these expensive phone bills. My most recent phone bill had been $395 for a month of long-distance calls to Austin.

In our discussion about getting married, we had to decide where we would live. Isidro agreed that we could get married in Chicago but asked if I would be willing to move to Austin to live with him in his apartment. We set our wedding date for September 15, 1995, because I thought it would be awesome to get married 45 years after my parents got married. However, after thinking about Harper's schedule, I didn't think it was fair for me to start the fall semester and then leave when I got married. Therefore, we decided to change the wedding date to July 1, 1995.

We continued to discuss why it would be better to live in Austin. He explained that he was concerned about his arthritis flaring up. It had been in remission and he didn't want the cold weather to affect it. I hated the cold winters in Chicago, and when I saw how beautiful it was in Austin when I was there for New Year's, I was sold on the idea that Austin would be a better place to live. However, I couldn't believe that I was leaving my life as I had always known it. First, I was going to leave a job that I loved. Second, and most difficult, I was going to leave my family. Still, with fear and all, I told Isidro we would live in Austin.

Everyone thought I was crazy. I didn't blame them. I thought it was a crazy decision too. Why did I decide to give up my life for a person I had seen three times in a matter of three months? The only explanation I could think of is that I felt that this was my destiny, and my gut told me it was the right thing to do. I told my mother, "Mom, remember Isidro? Well, I am going to marry him in six months." The first sentence that came out of her mouth was, "Mentiras; no puedes. (You are lying; you can't)." And then when I told her that I planned to move to Austin, that was too much for her and she couldn't continue the conversation—not because she was angry at me, but because she feared I had made a rash decision. I talked to Isidro that evening, and he said that he and his parents would come to Chicago during my spring break. He would officially ask for my hand in marriage so that my mom could become more comfortable with the idea.

Isidro and his parents arrived in March. Other than our wedding, the main topic of conversation was Selena Quintanilla's shooting and sudden death. In Texas, Selena was an icon and her death shook the state with sadness. We worked hard during the five-day visit and took care of important wedding details that needed both of our decisions. We secured the church and the banquet hall. In addition, Isidro gave me an engagement ring (which we ended up buying together). Because he was going back to Texas, all the wedding preparations were going to depend on me. The first thing I wanted to do was to inform Tom, my boss, about our decision and to give him notice so that he could find my replacement when I left.

CHAPTER 16

S tress consumed me for the following four months. I wasn't only taking care of all the preparations for the wedding, but I was also planning to leave my job and move to an entirely new state. I was also trying to convince my parents that everything was going to be alright. Looking back, I better understand all that they were feeling. On the one hand, they were happy for me because deep down, they hoped that someday I would start my own family. On the other hand, they were sad and worried because I was the child that needed most support and yet was the only one that was not going to live close to them like their other children. I tried to be sensitive to their concerns, but I was also very excited.

At first, my plan was to have twelve couples in my wedding party, which included all my siblings plus Isidro's four sisters. I thought that was already a huge wedding party, but before I knew it, the wedding party kept growing. So many people were excited for me. Gerardo, Daniel, Lucino, Sara, Shirley, plus a couple of other high school friends all ended up being in my wedding party. Soon after, cousins and other extended family wanted to participate. Once it was over twenty people, I said to myself, *Heck, why not. Let me include every niece and nephew in my wedding party too.* Every single person, all fifty bridesmaids, wore purple, my wedding color.

The invitations were perfect. I designed them with the slogan we had been chanting when we met: "Together United, We'll Never Be

Defeated." The most challenging part of my wedding preparations was my wedding dress. Lalo's wife Irene took me to several bridal shops, and I would always come home discouraged. The dresses were so heavy! I wanted to walk down the aisle on my crutches but feared tripping on the dress. Finally, I decided that the only option was to get the dress custom made. Irene found a seamstress who agreed to make my dress. It was great because she made it as light as possible with a removable train. I also struggled to find the appropriate shoes. I still wore my brace on my left side but wanted to find a nice shoe for my right foot. I knew that heels were out of the question, so I decided to buy a white canvas shoe and I adorned it myself with lace and dainty jeweled pieces. I also didn't want my crutches to steal the show and get all the attention, so I bought white satin fabric to wrap them with. I also wrapped Isidro's crutches with black satin fabric to match his tux.

Isidro was not only enthused about the wedding but also about the honeymoon. I'd told him about all the fun I'd had on the cruise with Sara, so we decided to go on a cruise to Mexico. We booked the cruise for a Monday, two days after our wedding. The cruise was only for five days because we planned to drive to Austin with all my possessions. My brother Lalo agreed to drive the U-Haul and help us settle down in Austin. My organizational skills were paramount for me to pull off such a huge wedding, plus a honeymoon and a move, all on my own, while still employed full time. I also organized for Isidro's family to stay at my siblings' homes so that they didn't have to incur the cost of a hotel when they came to the wedding.

July 1, 1995, ended up being a glorious day. I had feared extremely hot weather but was gifted with a beautiful sunny day in the low 80s. Isidro stayed at Lalo's house so that he wouldn't see me until we were at the church. I wasn't nervous, but after an unexpected incident, I became a nervous wreck. My hair was done, my dress was on, and my makeup was perfect. The photographer wanted to take some pictures of me getting ready. He saw the lipstick on my dresser so he grabbed it and asked me to pretend I was putting it on so he could take a picture. I put the tube right by my lips as he got near enough to take a close-up. Suddenly, the focus lens of his camera fell off, right onto my lipstick, causing it to slash a huge red mark down the front of my dress. I started to cry when I saw the red streak. Luckily, my mom had always been good under pressure. She told me to calm down and to take the dress off. I don't know what she did, but when she brought the dress back, the streak was gone. The photographer felt awful and ended up giving me a huge discount because of it.

I also became very sentimental when my parents gave me their blessing before heading to the church. I couldn't contain my tears. I loved them so much and felt so blessed for all they did for me to be successful and happy. I worried about them because I'd be leaving. Just as they supported me, I too had become their support by taking care of business when an English translator was needed. In addition, they were on a fixed income because my mother never worked, and my dad didn't receive much from social security. I had observed that they were slowing down, and I prayed for their health and well-being. I am certain they were going through a whole range of emotions as well. Here I was, about to get married and leave, after all the years of suffering. My mom gave me her blessing as she visibly fought her tears back. My dad also gave his blessing, but quietly—he couldn't talk or else he would have broken down crying.

Father John from Life Directions married Isidro and me on that magnificent day. The ceremony was beautiful, full of people who wished us happiness. Perhaps because of the lipstick incident, the photographer went out of his way to capture every moment of the beautiful day. He even asked a resident across from the church if he could go inside their home to the second floor so he could take a picture of the entire wedding party. We let go of balloons and afterward headed to my mom's house to wait until the reception. Originally, I had booked a park to take pictures in, but I thought my mom's garden was more beautiful than any park. My mom's love for her flowers was evident as the vibrant colors reflected off my white dress. I couldn't believe I was married.

I had told myself over and over, *Marriage is not for you.* No one ever told me that, but somehow, I always got that message. Interestingly, I never had considered marrying someone with a disability. But I knew Isidro was the right person for me and that is all that mattered. I thanked God for uniting me to a man that loved and accepted me exactly how I was. He didn't care that I wore different shoes or that I might fall when least expected. He loved me for who I was and for my values. Similarly, I saw past his disability and was able to admire his determination and how he didn't let his disability stop him. I loved him for his fortitude and his positive outlook on life. I had put all my hopes on him.

The reception was like a blur. Everyone was having fun, dancing, and celebrating our happiness. Everything ran like clockwork in terms of dinner and cutting the cake. The only glitch occurred during our first dance. We had chosen "Endless Love" by Lionel Richie, but the DJ put the cassette in the wrong direction so the song that started was "Penny Lover." We laughed about this for many years to come. We also danced the dollar dance, which is a common part of a Mexican wedding reception. The idea is that guests pin money on the dress or tuxedo to dance a few moments with the bride or groom. With a couple of my dancing companions, I was so emotional that I started to cry, but of course they were tears of happiness. I was a married woman at the age of thirty, and I was married to a man who completed me because he was able to do all the things I couldn't. I also completed him because I was able to do all the things he couldn't do in turn.

Our honeymoon was a five-day cruise to Mexico. We had a great time, though there were a couple of awkward moments. I noticed that Isidro was a big-time photographer and that he would take his time to get the best shot. At first, I was offended when he didn't want me in the picture when he was taking a picture of some site. I think he noticed that I was feeling hurt because soon after he started to include me in his pictures. I felt like I was on vacation with a stranger, but I suppose that every new couple feels the same, especially when there had been no prior intimacy until the honeymoon. I did enjoy getting some time to relax since the previous months had been so full of stress.

After our honeymoon, we flew back to Chicago and planned to drive toward Austin the next day. Lalo already had picked up the U-Haul and packed it with all my things plus all the wedding gifts we had received. He was going to drive the U-Haul and follow my Cavalier which Isidro and I would be driving. Although I knew that I loved Isidro and that he loved me, saying farewell to my parents was so difficult. Isidro went out with Lalo to return his tuxedo, so I had time with my parents alone. I took an envelope out of my purse that I had prepared. I gave it to my dad and said, "Dad, don't worry about me. Here is ten thousand dollars that I have saved. I want you to keep it for me. In the event things don't work out, I know you will welcome me with open arms, and I will have some money to start me off." My dad said, "Do you fear something isn't going to work out?" I said, "No; I've just learned to be prepared for anything. I learned that from you." He smiled and put the envelope in his pocket and said, "The money will be here for whenever you need it."

My parents were understandably sad and worried about my move. I reassured them and told them Isidro promised to take good care of me. My mom said, "I know. He will keep his promise." I hugged each of them tightly and said, "You can visit, and we will visit too." They didn't respond, but just hugged me tighter. I know my mom's heart was breaking, but she never shed a tear in front of me. She had always been tough for the both of us. My happiness was not complete because I was leaving the two people that I loved most in the world.

We took off to Austin early the next day and drove straight through. We drove slowly because we didn't want to lose each other. When we arrived, the temperature was unbearably hot. Isidro took us to his apartment, which was in a quiet cul-de-sac in Austin. The apartment was on the ground level and had a handicapped parking space right in front. Lalo immediately began bringing everything in. Isidro gave us a tour and I was surprised that, although it was not a big place, it had ample room for both of us. The space included a nice bedroom with a queen-sized bed, a large bathroom with a walk-in shower, and a combined living room/dining room next to a small kitchen. We had decided that I would just move into the home for the time being so that we could save money to purchase our own home.

Lalo was sweating profusely and asked Isidro, "How do we turn on the air conditioner?" Isidro stood up to turn on his ceiling fan and responded, "This fan cools pretty good, so I never needed an AC." My brother was in shock and he said, "I am not leaving my sister in this hell. Let's go to Walmart and buy at least a window AC." I was concerned that Isidro would be insulted, but he laughed and said, "Yeah, I guess I am used to this heat, but she isn't." My brother bought a window air conditioner and installed it. He also put many of the gifts where we directed him to put them. He had to leave the next day, so he worked hard to get me settled.

After Lalo returned the U-Haul and we took him to the airport, Isidro and I went to the H-E-B supermarket, which we didn't have in Chicago. We purchased groceries since Isidro was going back to work the following day. I also purchased their newspapers so that I could begin looking for jobs. I was hoping to find a job at either Austin Community College or University of Texas. While searching for jobs, I also dedicated myself to cleaning the apartment. Although I was impressed at how tidy Isidro kept his house, I did notice some tendencies to clean superficially. Every day, I would clean something and wait for him to figure out what I did.

Days were passing by, and although I had sent resumes, I wasn't getting any calls. I continued my cleaning frenzy. I thought I would surprise him by cleaning an old wooden desk that seemed cluttered to me. I took my time and made sure to organize it without throwing out anything that seemed important. I saw a brown paper bag full of coins that included quarters, dimes, nickels, and pennies. I thought to myself, *Poor Isidro, he probably doesn't even remember about this change.* I had seen a Chase bank around the corner, so I took the bag of change and cashed it out. I was happy to know that it was over a hundred dollars. I was surely going to surprise him!

When he got home, I proudly said, "Here." I handed him the money I had received in exchange for his coins. He was puzzled and asked, "What is this?" I said, "Well, it's technically your money, but I bet you didn't know you had it." I said, "I found all the coins in your desk and took them to the bank." His eyes opened wide and said, "You did what?" I repeated what I had said but now wasn't sure I should be proud. He said, "That was my coin collection. I had coins there probably worth a lot of money." I couldn't believe it. What had I done? He noticed that I was getting visibly upset, so he took a deep breath and said, "Don't worry; it's not a big deal. I should've told you." After how he handled that situation, I knew we would make it.

During my job search time, while Isidro went to work, I tried not to venture too far. I cooked, baked, and cleaned. I had seen a few insects here and there, mostly by the bathroom or front door. But one day, I was cooking dinner and I saw the biggest, most gross-looking bug ever. I almost dropped the dish I had in my hands. I was petrified of bugs and never dared to kill them. I was alone, so my only hope was that it would go and hide. My nerves were on edge and I stared at the darn bug most of the afternoon. It finally disappeared and I sighed a sigh of relief.

When Isidro came home, I told him about the bug. We looked for the huge pest, but it never came out of hiding. It came out again the next day, though, when I was alone once again. This continued for a couple of weeks until Isidro was beginning to think I was making it up. I even hired my sisters-in-law's kids to hunt for it. They made good money, but the bug never showed its face. Isidro bought some bug repellent that we sprayed around the house. Still, the bug would come out whenever it was just the two of us. It started to be a contest between me and that humongous gross thing. It was hard to believe that I had survived polio, twelve surgeries, and eight broken bones, but I was at the mercy of this insect.

It was such a relief when I found a job. Unfortunately, it wasn't at either of the colleges because there were no positions available for working with students with disabilities. I was hired by United Cerebral Palsy (UCP) to help with a new grant they had received where individuals could apply to have their homes modified for access. My title was Housing Counselor and my responsibility was to make four visits per day to the homes of applicants to see if they qualified. At first, I was concerned if I would be able to do the job, but soon I discovered it was the perfect job. I figured, if I can't enter the home, then the house is inaccessible, and they qualify for the grant. It was very taxing on me, and it was exhausting to constantly be getting in and out of my car. At least I learned the city well because I drew a map of how to get to each visit. The pay wasn't great since it was a not-for-profit organization, but it helped that the cost of living in Texas was lower.

Our relationship was solid, but I was unhappy because I missed my family so much. I learned that Isidro's family was different and not as unified as mine. I worried about my parents and how they were dealing with my absence. I would watch our wedding video and sob when I saw everyone I loved so much. I think I played the wedding video a thousand times just to see my parents and the rest of the family. I also wondered if Isidro and I would ever be parents. I knew that if we lived in Austin, I couldn't dream of that because I'd lack the type of support I needed. Some days, sadness overtook me. I was sad not only because I missed my family, but also because my disability frustrated me more than ever. For example, as a new wife, I broke all my drinking glasses, and though I had a brand-new box that my brother had stored on the top cabinet, I was not able to get it down and there was no one I could ask.

Additionally, though I imagined that the weather in Austin was better than the snowy, cold Chicago, I had a difficult time with the humidity and extreme heat. I was so glad Lalo had bought me the air conditioner. Also, to my surprise, I felt more discriminated against being Mexican than ever before. Although people had the same skin color I did, they didn't view themselves as Mexicans or Latinos. They would stress that they were Texan-Americans. On several occasions, I was corrected on how I pronounced street names, like Guadalupe and Manchaca, when I was certain I knew how to pronounce them. And, I couldn't find the Mexican products that I needed to cook the many dishes I had learned from my mom.

Isidro was patient and tried to make me happy any way he could. He knew I loved Los Bukis and when he found out they would be playing in town, he bought tickets for us to attend the concert. We both went in wheelchairs because otherwise we would be more likely to fall in the big crowds. When we got in, I saw a security guard and asked if there was a better place for Isidro and me to sit so that we could watch the concert. The security guard didn't speak English so then I repeated my question in Spanish. He got all excited and in Spanish asked me, "Can you help me translate something into English?" I said, "Sure." He told me to tell this other tall security guard that no one should be allowed to get on the stage.

Once I finished translating all the directions, he said, "Come, I am taking you where you can see the concert better." He took us backstage, and I was able to personally meet Marco Antonio Solis, the main singer, and take pictures with the group. In fact, I even had to use the bathroom in their dressing room because it was the only accessible bathroom backstage. The musicians were shocked when I came out of a stall. Everyone who knows me knows that meeting Marco Antonio Solis was a dream come true. So, Austin turned out not to be so bad.

Unbeknownst to me, Isidro was working on a plan to allow us to move back to Chicago. He talked to his employer, JCPenney, and asked about the possibility of transferring to Chicago. He saw how unhappy I was, and when he heard that he could transfer and have a job, he gave me the good news. He said, "Let's move to Chicago." I said, "But what about your arthritis?" He said, "We can try it and see how it goes." I couldn't believe what I was hearing. I then gave him a surprise as well. I said, "When we move, we can buy our own place."

He looked at me and said, "Remember, we are saving for a down payment." I then told him about the ten thousand dollars my dad was keeping for me. We were both so excited and full of happiness.

Harper had sought to replace me, but their search had failed. I was still in contact with Juanita, and she was keeping me informed. When they posted the search again, I applied for the same position I had left. I had no idea if I would get the position, but regardless, we were going to be moving back to Chicago to live. Harper selected to interview me yet again, so they paid for me to fly home. Isidro took some vacation and accompanied me. I knew everyone on the search committee, but I took it very seriously and didn't assume it was a given that I would be hired. I even asked Joan and Tom to write letters of recommendations in the event I didn't get the Harper job and had to look for another position somewhere else. However, after the interview, it was fun to show everyone my wedding pictures.

After I got back to Texas, Joan, the Dean of Student Development, called me while I was at work at UCP. She offered me the position at Harper at the same salary I had left. The only hitch was that I would have to go through the tenure process all over again. But still, I was ecstatic! I gave my two-weeks' notice at UCP and, because I had connected well with my team, we had a farewell picnic. Even though I'd only been with UCP for seven months, we had all become friends. They couldn't believe that I would be making more than double what we were getting paid. I knew that my friends from UCP had been in one of my life's chapters, but that I probably wouldn't ever see them again.

Packing to go home was easy. We decided to leave everything behind and just take our clothes and our personal belongings. Isidro and I were about to take a leap of faith but knew my family would be there to help us out. When I gave my parents the news, they became so excited. It had been ten months since I had left and, though my parents never missed sending me their blessings from afar, they couldn't help but miss my presence as much as I missed theirs. They welcomed us with open arms to move into the little apartment I had set up before leaving so that Isidro and I could have our privacy. Isidro had a Ford Ranger pickup that he brought to Chicago for a mode of transportation. Mon and Lalo went to Austin to help us with the move. We packed up my red Cavalier and Isidro's truck and headed home to the place that would always be there for me no matter what.

On the long road trip from Austin to Chicago, I had time to reflect. The ten months in Austin had been very difficult for me, but I was convinced that moving had been the best decision. Now I was certain that Isidro and I could make it on our own. With our respective disabilities, we'd managed to live a normal life. If I had not moved, I would have always wondered if I could make it on my own. I'd matured and learned more than ever during those ten months away. I learned how to best connect with Isidro, and we grew to understand each other better than I ever thought we could. I looked forward to our future life together.

CHAPTER 17

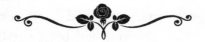

My parents welcomed us home after our long drive from Austin. I was scheduled to begin work the first week of June, so I had a week to get situated. The first thing we wanted to do was to look for a realtor to help us purchase our first home. We decided to look for a condo near where we both were going to work. Reyna knew of a realtor who could help us go see the homes. For obvious reasons, we needed a first-floor condo with accessibility. We were fortunate to find a nice condo in Palatine not too long after we got back. The condo was on the first floor and it had an attached garage. We ended up living with my parents for only one month; the closing was fast due to our great credit and the fact that we already had the down payment. We needed basic furniture since we left everything in Austin, so my sister Reyna looked for the best deals.

Our new home was beautiful and luxurious. The condo had two bedrooms, two baths, with a spacious living room/dining room. The kitchen was quaint, making it very convenient for me because I could sit on a stool and reach almost everything while I cooked. The master bedroom had its own bathroom with a sunken Whirlpool bathtub. I was so looking forward to soaking away the stress any time I needed it. The condo complex was new construction, so it had brand new white carpet in the living room and dining room. Moving in didn't take a long time since we didn't have any large furniture to move, and when we bought furniture, we had it delivered. My sister Reyna lived close to us, so she was always just a call away from coming to help us with anything we needed.

We started our American middle-class life. We would go to work and, in the evenings, figure out dinner and work on our own things. On the weekends, we would go to the movies, out to dinner, and of course to see my parents or attend any family events that were happening. We kept our home organized and clean since we both took pride in our beautiful home. We didn't often have company at the beginning, but as I got reacquainted with work, I started to create programming to support the students. Before all the policies with boundaries with students existed, I had study groups come to my home. My students connected very well with me and were very appreciative of the open-door policy I had for them. I wanted the students to succeed and did whatever I could so that could happen.

My students showed their appreciation in unique ways with unexpected gifts. At the end of the semesters, especially around the holiday break, students would present their gifts. I remember several of the most unique ones. One student had the gift all wrapped up and said, "Open it. It is my gift for all the help you give me." I responded, "Thank you, but you don't need to give me gifts." I slowly opened the gift and tried to figure out what it was. Turns out it was a Flowbee home haircutting system. The Flowbee needed to be connected to a vacuum cleaner, and then the hair that was cut from the razor would be sucked in. I was keeping my hair short at that time, and the student thought I could save money that way. Another gift that left me confused was a George Foreman Grill. Maybe the student thought using a regular grill was too dangerous for me?

After three good evaluations, I received tenure again. I loved my job, and Tom was giving me more responsibilities. He trusted my opinion about the direction of our department. We went through the process of changing the department's name from Center for Students with Disabilities to Access and Disability Services (ADS). The change was to be inclusive of the Deaf population that didn't view their inability to hear as a disability but considered themselves to be a part of a culture. The number of our students was increasing and now included new populations. Many students were now being diagnosed with Attention Deficit Disorder and other psychological disabilities. Tom supported the staff in learning as much as we could about these conditions. This gave me an opportunity to travel to different parts of the United States to attend conferences of the national organization that focused on colleges and universities. Association of Higher Education and Disability (AHEAD) gave us the most up-to-date information so we could return to our workplace with new ideas.

I also continued to be active with Life Directions. I wasn't attending their Focus Life weekend retreats anymore, but I hosted Life Directions Circle discussions where we would read and discuss scripture. Two of the people who attended these meetings became very good friends and they started to hang around with me and Isidro socially. We would order pizza and play board games or just talk. They felt that my home was comfortable and cozy. Sometimes I would make a Mexican dish and they would rant and rave about how well I cooked. Isidro and I were content with our lifestyle, but we still wondered if we would be able to handle raising children. Though we did our best to fill our voids, I think we both still felt that something was missing.

After three years of marriage, I started to ask myself, *Now what? Is this what my life will be like until I die?* I hated that I always wanted more. It seemed to me that I was always looking for ways to bring more stress into my life. After all, I was already living beyond what anyone had expected for me. Who would have believed that the dirty little girl crawling around in the dirt in La Purísima would someday have a career and be married? Was I crazy for always wanting more? No matter how often I would contemplate all my blessings, I continued with my desire to form my own family and have children. I had researched polio and rheumatoid arthritis and knew that neither would affect our offspring genetically, so I justified my desire. I went for a medical checkup, as did Isidro, and we were healthy except for our respective disabilities. Together, Isidro and I made the decision to pursue having children.

We didn't have to try too long before I found out I was pregnant. I was so very happy! I went for a medical examination to confirm my pregnancy and was given the exciting news that not only was I pregnant, but he had seen *two* little hearts on the ultrasound. Wow, two babies? I was worried about being able to care for one baby and never imagined two. I was still flabbergasted, and Isidro and I gave my parents the good news. I knew that as I started to show, I probably would have to use my wheelchair more often, which I was already starting to do anyway. The active job in Austin, going to four visits a day, had strained my ankle and good knee, and now I was experiencing more pain than ever. I started noticing that I couldn't walk as far or stand as long before becoming extremely exhausted. I knew I would have to figure this out when the time came.

My exuberant feeling didn't last long. I had been scheduled for a follow-up appointment two weeks after I was given the terrific news, and when I went, I had another ultrasound. The doctor had said that he would probably do more ultrasounds than customary just to make sure everything was progressing. He was unsure if my curved spine would affect the pregnancy. As the doctor did the ultrasound, Isidro and I noticed his expression change. He kept rubbing my stomach with the instrument in all directions. After a couple of minutes of sliding through the gooey liquid, he put his instrument down. He said, "I have some bad news." Isidro and I just looked at him, waiting for him to continue. He said, "It appears that the two heartbeats are not beating any longer." My jaw dropped. I couldn't believe this was happening to us. He went on to say, "Don't worry. Many women have miscarriages and then are fine with future pregnancies." I started to cry but was speechless. He said, "This is the body's way of protecting you from pregnancies that started off wrong." I didn't care to listen to his explanation. He told me that I could have a procedure to take the missed pregnancy or I could just wait for it to naturally happen. I decided on the latter.

Besides going through the physical turmoil and our own emotional pain, it was so difficult to tell my mom and the rest of the family. I was so upset and didn't want anyone to try to console me. I wasn't much in the mood to socialize, so I immersed myself in my job. I started presenting in classes and teaching faculty and staff about disabilities. I started to form professional relationships with faculty and staff outside of my department. I wanted to focus on what I was good at and on ways that my disability didn't matter.

The doctor had been right. Two months later, I found out I was pregnant again. This time, Isidro and I decided to keep it to ourselves, though it was very difficult not to tell my mom. We ended up being glad, because once again, I had a miscarriage in the tenth week of the pregnancy. I was so afraid that my disability was causing my losses. This time, the doctor described, "This was an ectopic pregnancy that needed to be terminated because the fertilized egg is not in the uterus." I didn't care to know the specific scientific explanation. All I knew is that, again, I was pregnant one day and the next I was no longer having a baby. This time I did have to go through a procedure to dispel my pregnancy. It was even difficult to watch TV because the news was constantly reporting on the story of a mom in Iowa who'd had septuplets on the same day I had my procedure.

Devastated and wanting to forget what had happened, I continued working hard and volunteering with Life Directions. I kept telling myself that I couldn't have everything, that I should just appreciate the good man I had. Isidro was going through his own emotions. We didn't like discussing what had happened, so his approach was just to try to get me to forget. He also worked extra hours and tried to drown his sorrows watching sports. I lacked peace because I was angry at God. I couldn't understand how he could allow one woman who already had a child to have seven babies when I was not granted even one. I couldn't understand God's plan in all of this. I was angry for a long time.

At the beginning of 1997, I was given the news that I was pregnant for the third time. But I didn't even allow myself to become excited. It was as if I already knew the fate of the pregnancy. I still followed the doctor's instructions and began to take the prenatal vitamins. I was quite familiar with all the steps. Even when we went to the ultrasound and heard the baby's heart, I remained cautiously optimistic. The doctor had told me that, once the first trimester is done, the danger is usually over. After completing the first trimester, I started to feel a little bit of hope and excitement. I told my family that I was pregnant and had just passed the first trimester. Because of my fear of falling while walking on my braces and crutches, I decided to use my wheelchair more regularly.

My pregnancy and being in a wheelchair presented a whole new challenge in driving. Typically, after I parked my car, I walked to my office and then would use the wheelchair that I'd left there. However, with winter coming, I didn't even want to take that walk anymore to avoid the chance of falling. But I was not strong enough to lift my chair to put it in my trunk either. I researched and found out about a mechanical device that would fold and lift the wheelchair to the rooftop of the car. It was exactly what I needed. This way, all I would have to do was transfer onto my driver seat, and then use the operating handle to have the wheelchair lifted.

It was not an easy time. I was constantly worrying and thinking something was wrong. Any time I felt even the tiniest of pains, I started to panic. I wanted this pregnancy so badly that it consumed every waking moment, and even my sleep as well.

The first week of May, I had a doctor's visit. I was now nineteen weeks along, so the doctor was very positive that things would work out. After my exam, he concluded everything was looking good and that the baby seemed strong and healthy. I chose not to know the gender since I wanted to be surprised at his or her birth. I left the doctor's office and, for the first time, I felt positive and thought, *I am going to be a mom soon.* I couldn't remember the last time I had been so happy. We went out to celebrate that we would soon be parents.

On my birthday, May 17, I was awakened by a sharp pain in my abdomen. I let it pass and stayed still, hoping that I wouldn't feel it again. It was a Saturday, and we had planned to sleep in, visit my parents, and in the evening go to a fancy dinner to celebrate my special day. Isidro was still sound asleep, so I just laid there quietly. About ten minutes later, I had the same awful pain. This time, I moved Isidro to wake him up. I said, "Babe, I have a pain right here," pointing to the exact location of my pain. He said, "Maybe you slept in a bad position. Why don't you move to a different position?" As I did that, I felt relief. I didn't feel the pain again for the rest of the day. We decided to cancel our plans and just stay in bed resting.

By the next day, though, we became more alarmed because the pain came back. Now it was so sharp that it brought tears to my eyes. We decided to call the doctor early that morning. Because it was Sunday, the answering service took the call and the nurse asked me to describe the pain. She said, "It might be best for you to go to the ER at Lutheran General Hospital to be checked out." We hung up the phone and I got ready to go to the hospital.

Isidro got me to the hospital as fast as he could. We were taken to the maternity ward right away. I was given a robe and was examined by the doctor on call. Isidro and I couldn't talk because we were both equally scared. We didn't know what to say so we both remained speechless. The doctor said, "I am going to go call your doctor, and I will be right back." He left the room and I knew then that something was terribly wrong. I started to sob. Isidro stood up and came by my bed, caressing my hair and just remained quiet. Deep down, I think he also knew that this was not a good sign.

My actual doctor came to examine me later in the morning. After he examined me, he said, "The pain you had are contractions. You have started to dilate and because you are only 19 weeks pregnant, we must prolong the pregnancy if we can." He shared his plan to invert my bed so my head would lean down and my feet would be on top in an attempt to push the baby back and stop the premature labor. I was miserable and in excruciating pain. Because of my severe scoliosis, usually I slept almost in a sitting position and couldn't lay flat because of the pain. I was crying and felt I was being tortured. Isidro didn't know what to do so he called my mom to tell her what was happening. The doctors didn't want to give me pain medication because of the baby, so all I could do was be brave.

As I lay inverted, the memories of all my past pain came to me. I was angry that God had been so harsh to me. I was livid that no matter how hard I worked to overcome each challenge, God would allow me to continue suffering and make my life so difficult. I wondered if I was being punished for something but couldn't figure what. I always tried to be positive, help others, and be a faithful Christian. I remembered that my mom had always told me that life was a valley of tears and felt that she was right. How come God didn't show me any mercy? I cried enough tears to fill a valley myself. I spent all night in agony and was disheartened when I was told that I might be in this position for weeks. I doubted my ability to resist and felt guilty for wanting relief regardless of the consequences. This was not the birthday weekend I had expected.

The next day, my mom came to the hospital with my sister-in-law Irene. They tried to console me and tell me that putting me in this position would help. I just cried. I didn't even know the source of my tears any longer. Was I crying out of pain? Was I crying because I knew I was never going to be a mom? Was I crying because of how hard my life had been? Was I crying because I felt beaten by what I felt was stronger than me? Perhaps it was all those reasons combined into an endless flow of tears.

The doctor came to examine me in the afternoon of May 19. He looked disappointed and said, "This has not helped. You are still seven centimeters dilated." To examine me, the doctor had raised my bed, so I was breathing a sigh of relief. The horrendous painful pressure on my spine had been lessened by raising the bed. My back pain had decreased with the simple change of position. I asked, "So the time I stayed upside down didn't help?" He said, "Well, you are still dilated, so you are still in danger of having a premature birth." He continued with the bad news and said, "If you give birth, there is no way the baby can survive this early." Barely able to talk, I said, "So now what?" He said, "Let me talk to my partners and see if they think we can stitch you to hold the baby back." I knew that wouldn't be good, but I still preferred that to being put upside down again.

At about 10 PM, I started to have severe pain again and went into full labor. I was quickly taken to a delivery room. The contractions were coming every minute, and they were strong. The doctor said that I was about to give birth and directed me to push. At 11 PM, I gave birth to a little boy. I was exhausted but was able to see him for a moment as they took him to another table to clean him up. They asked if I wanted to see him. I nodded yes, so they brought him over to me. My mom and sister-in-law were sobbing, trying to console me. My mom was praying out loud asking for God to help me for losing my baby. We all assumed that he was born without life. I looked down at him and saw how big he was. His skin was dark and very transparent, allowing me to see through to his veins. I cried as I saw him, when suddenly I saw his little chest rise. I felt guilty because he scared me. I yelled, "He is not dead." At first, the nurse said, "No, I am sorry, but he is not alive." Just as she said that, we saw his little chest expand again. This time, the nurse didn't say anything and quickly took my baby.

Shortly after, the doctor told me that he was barely alive but that there was nothing they could do to help him live. My mom said, "We need to baptize him. Ask him if they can send a priest." I asked the doctor, who said that he would send a chaplain right away. I held my baby as the chaplain baptized him. We had selected a boy's name long before, so we decided to name him Cristian. Using a tiny seashell, the chaplain poured a bit of water on his forehead, baptizing him while he was faintly breathing. The chaplain mentioned that he was going to request a social security number for him as part of a live-birth procedure.

It was so painful to see my mom in such despair. She pleaded to God to help me. She asked, "Why do you send this pain to her? Send it to me, not her." I just held Cristian, and I baptized him again with my tears of goodbye. Just when I said hello, I was also saying goodbye. He gave his last breath at 1:00 AM on May 20, just two hours after his birth. Isidro and I mourned the loss of our son, but I didn't realize that my mom mourned not only the loss of her grandson but the pain of seeing me suffer in this most tormenting way. If anyone could understand me, I was sure she did. She had suffered the same pain when everyone thought I was going to die.

A very kind nurse took some pictures of Cristian with a Polaroid camera and asked me if I wanted better pictures. She volunteered to bring in a digital camera and take better quality shots. I thanked her but wasn't even sure I would want to see his pictures. The doctor came to my room and examined me. In trying to console me, he said words that I never forgot. He said, "Ms. Herrera, I am sorry for your loss, but your body is just not made for babies." I burst out in tears. I thought to myself, *Not only did I lose my son, but it's my fault.* The doctor got nervous as I cried and said that I could be discharged as soon as I felt well enough. I told him I wanted to go home as soon as possible. He signed my discharge papers, and I was brought paperwork to complete before going home. One of the forms asked what my wishes were regarding Cristian's remains. Another asked if I wanted an autopsy performed. I indicated that I didn't since I already knew why he had died. He was simply too premature.

It was Memorial Day weekend when I was discharged and sent home. Because of the holidays, the funeral home didn't have access to Cristian until afterward. Isidro and I were drained so we decided to get away to Wisconsin Dells, just three hours away. We didn't want to be consoled; we wanted to be alone with our pain. As we were packing to leave, my doctor called. I answered the phone and he said, "Ms. Herrera, I am calling to ask for your permission to do an autopsy on your son." I responded, "No. I don't want that. I indicated that on the form." He insisted and said, "But we can get valuable information that could help us determine the cause of his death." I replied in an angry tone, "I already know why he died. He was too premature because of my body." I started crying and when Isidro saw this, he took away the phone to talk to the doctor. As I walked to my room, I heard him reiterate that we didn't want the autopsy.

Just as we were about to walk out of our condo, the phone rang again. I said, "I hope it isn't the doctor again." I answered. This time it was the nice nurse who took the only pictures we had of Cristian.

She said, "Ms. Herrera, did your doctor call?" Frustrated about the issue of the autopsy, I said, "Yes, he did." She quickly said, "Oh good. I just felt awful that I couldn't take pictures of Cristian because when I went, they had already taken him for an autopsy." I said, "What?" She repeated the same thing but in different words and said, "I tried to take pictures, but I was too late because they had performed an autopsy on him." I said, "The doctor called to ask for my permission to have the autopsy done. Are you saying that they did one even when I said no?" She cleared her throat knowing that she had said something that compromised the doctor and said, "I just wanted to say sorry for not taking more pictures." She quickly excused herself and said goodbye before I could stop her from hanging up.

I remember that weekend getaway as one of the darkest times of my life. Everyone was out and about, as happy as could be. I questioned how people could be so happy. I felt as if I was the only one who knew how awful life could be. I didn't feel like eating, talking, or anything. All I wanted to do was cry. The only break from my sadness was when I would get a surge of anger. I asked myself, *How could the doctor do what he did? How could he try to deceive me by asking for permission for something that had already been done?* Deep inside me, I knew that I would have forgiven the doctor if he had called to apologize and explain that a mistake had been made. However, I couldn't forget that he knowingly tried to deceive me! I wasn't willing to forgive him for that. Thinking about the incident consumed my every thought. I was so angry. Angry at God for being so cruel, angry at myself for wanting to have everything and causing Cristian's death because of my messed-up body, and angry at the doctor for being so cold and deceitful to me when I was most in despair. I knew that I would never be the same again. This time, I wouldn't be able to recover and move on as I had often done.

The more we talked to family and friends, the more that I was certain that I had to seek justice for Cristian. When we got back home from the Dells, we went to pick up Cristian's ashes. The funeral home put them in a little heart-shaped ceramic box. I didn't know that such a tiny item would bring so much pain. I felt that no one could understand my pain, not even Isidro. I knew he was hurting, but I also believed it was a different pain than mine. I didn't go to family events and even struggled going to my parents' home. I felt that I was a reminder of something very painful for my mother. I started noticing that I was distancing myself from the people that I loved most.

That summer, I decided to attend the AHEAD conference in Las Vegas. Isidro decided to accompany me, thinking that it might be helpful to go to the city where we met for the first time. Tom and his wife Barbara also attended. After the day of conference sessions, Tom, Barbara, Isidro, and I decided to go to dinner. I was still very sad, but I was enjoying the distractions of the city. After we ate, we took the tram back to our hotel, the Mirage. I was using my wheelchair because the multiple pregnancies had really weakened me. I didn't feel safe to walk any more. I noticed that a stranger wearing a turban on his head was having a conversation with Isidro while they sat in the back of the tram. I was not close enough to distinguish what they were talking about. When we arrived at the Mirage, I got off with the rest of my companions as well as the stranger. Isidro yelled out, "Cuali, hold on. This man can help us!" Tom and Barbara went ahead while I waited for Isidro and the man.

Isidro excitedly said, "He can help us so we can have children." I felt aggravated immediately, thinking that Isidro had divulged private information. Isidro continued, "He knows about Cristian and how you can't have children." Angrily I said, "Why are you sharing our private life?" The man just stood there observing both of us without saying a word. "No, I didn't tell him anything. He knew it already." With this comment, the man felt he had the permission to talk. He said, "I know a lot about you." I smirked and said, "Oh yeah, like what?" He said, "I know you are very incredulous, that you sleep with seven pillows, that your father was an alcoholic, and that you will live a long and very difficult life." Scolding Isidro I said, "Why did you tell him all that?" Isidro quickly responded, "I didn't. He has powers, and he says he can help us so we can have a baby." I didn't know what to say, so I just stayed silent. The man's piercing look gave me chills. The man said, "For a hundred dollars, I can create a potion that will cure all the issues with bearing children." I gave him a skeptical look and told Isidro, "I am leaving and going up to my room." Isidro stayed behind talking to the man.

In bed Isidro shared that he had agreed that the man could call us at 7 AM the next day so that we could meet him and get the potion in exchange for the hundred dollars. All night, I was sleepless thinking about that mysterious guy. I drilled Isidro to see if he'd inadvertently told him anything about me. Isidro denied sharing anything with him, insisting that I should be more trusting. He said, "A hundred dollars is well worth it to try." I said, "Heck no, I am not going to drink anything. If you want to, you go ahead." Tired from the day, Isidro just turned around and fell asleep.

I started to freak out as he snored away. I wondered if, using his supposed powers, he knew where we lived. I couldn't believe that he knew how I slept and much less that my dad had been an alcoholic. I then started to worry that the guy knew where we were staying and might follow us to hurt us. I kept thinking the worst and couldn't take my anxiety anymore. I woke up Isidro and said, "Isidro, I don't want to meet that guy. I am scared." Half asleep, Isidro said, "Don't worry." I raised my voice and asked, "How do you want me not to worry when he knew so much about me?"

Now that we were both awake, I suggested that we let Tom know about the guy's proposal so that he would be aware in case something happened to us. It was almost 6 AM and I knew that Tom always mentioned being an early bird. I called his room and told him how scared I was. Within twenty minutes, both Tom and Barbara came into our room. I told them the whole experience in detail, stressing that I was very scared. Barbara had brought her Bible and she read a couple of verses trying to calm me down.

In a nutshell, they explained that there might be people who have the skill to read clues and figure out the past but that anyone who honestly wanted to help would never ask for money. I told them I didn't want anything from him and that I didn't know what we should do because he was going to call our room soon to arrange a meeting by the casino. Barbara said, "Don't worry, I will answer the call when the phone rings." Shortly afterward, the phone rang and Barbara said, "Hi, my friends here are Christian believers and don't believe in anything that doesn't come from Jesus. Please don't call again." She didn't give the other person an opportunity for a rebuttal before hanging up the phone. I thanked her but insisted that I wouldn't be in peace if I was at a hotel where he knew I was. They were such great friends that, without any judgment, they helped us move to a different hotel and even moved with us as well. I knew then that Tom and Barbara were real friends and not just my boss and his wife.

Back at home, I tried to alleviate my heartache; I worked harder than ever. I pushed hard to get promoted. I took all types of classes to earn the credits I needed for an early promotion. I enrolled in one course on substance abuse offered by Northern Illinois University. There were about twenty students enrolled, and during the introductions I learned that another Harper employee was taking the class. It felt reassuring to know that I had a colleague in the class. I had never met Bill, an adjunct, part-time faculty counselor in the Academic Advising and Counseling Center, but I was immediately able to connect with him. He reminded me of Santa Claus with his whitening beard and hair.

During lunch, I approached him and introduced myself. We ate lunch together, and I noticed he drank two twenty-ounce bottles of soda in thirty minutes. He must have been welcoming, because I opened up to him with personal information, such as my three pregnancies, that I would normally not share. When I told him about my recent loss, his eyes got wide with shock. I don't think he was prepared for that level of revelation. To ease the tension I was feeling, the only thing that came to mind was to joke with him. However, what was supposed to be a joke ended up being a total intrusion. I said, "Bill, you sure like soda. Be careful because too much soda may cause a bladder infection." He smiled and said, "I will remember that."

As part of the class, for one of the assignments we had to find a partner to do research and a presentation to the class on the topic of alcoholism. Bill and I decided to pair up and do a presentation on alcoholism among individuals with disabilities. We divided the tasks, and I was happy to discover that Bill was the research-type student, unlike me. We worked on a PowerPoint presentation, and I am sure he was concerned because I admitted that I had not read the bunch of articles he had sent me. I explained that I like to relate to the audience and use my personal experiences when I presented. I said, "Bill, don't worry. I will be ready to do my part of the presentation. Trust me."

On the day of the presentation, I brought props, which surprised Bill. I saw his continued worry! He probably was concerned and thought it shouldn't be a show-and-tell kind of presentation. He was stuck with me, though, and I smiled, hoping that he would trust me. He did his part of the presentation, giving statistics and the research he had found. When he was done, I took out my props, which were my wedding albums, and started passing them out. I started my part with, "Now that Bill has gone over the statistics of how alcoholism affects individuals with disabilities, let me tell you a true story. A person at my wedding party, my husband's friend Roy, died recently because of alcohol abuse."

I shared how Roy, who was a quadriplegic, died when he drank too much. I explained that he passed out and asphyxiated himself, although his friends thought he had just fallen asleep with his head down. Because of his level of alcohol consumption and his disability, he probably was unable to lift his head, which prevented him from being able to breathe. I had the class's full attention, and everyone enjoyed listening to the story and especially seeing my wedding pictures. They were amazed that I had fifty couples in the wedding party and that Roy had been part of it. Bill was in shock that my strategy worked and that we had earned an A in the assignment and for the class. Twenty years later, he hasn't allowed me to forget how I wooed the professor and students with hardly doing any work.

Bill and I became immediate friends, so much so that we had the privilege of working together in disability services when a full-time position opened. Although he wasn't a jolly Santa Claus but rather a bit sarcastic and crabby with me, still today, he is one of my best friends at Harper. We not only worked together but have spent many happy, fun moments going to various casinos. We refer to the casinos as special conferences where we exercise our fingers when playing the slot machines. We always tease each other, and I know others find our banter hilarious. However, even with all our bickering, we know we can always count on each other for anything.

Nothing alleviated the pain of losing Cristian, though. Isidro and I decided that we couldn't go through this experience again and would have to come to terms with it by being the best aunt and uncle instead. I hated to admit it, but it was so painful for me to see Rique's new baby girl, Jennifer, who was born the year after in October. I was happy for them, but I couldn't help asking, *Why me?* Jennifer was beautiful, but she was also a reminder of the son that I couldn't have. I saw how my parents adored her and felt guilty for my feelings of jealousy. I tried not to feel this way, but my pain was so raw. This had been even more painful than when I lost Mama Petra. The only thing that was beginning to help me mitigate the pain was writing. I started to write poems to express my pain. Poems like these were my salvation:

Broken Dreams

Life Began,
Baby Held,
Life Ended,
Goodbyes Said,
Tears Shed,
Dreams Gone,
Nightmares Come,
Sacrifices Wasted,
Faith Questioned,
Time Passes,
Acceptance Comes.

Hidden Pain

People think my pain is gone,
After all, a month has passed by.
Four weeks ago, I had and lost a son,
But even today, I still cry and cry.

It isn't the first time I've shed tears,
For I've suffered a lot throughout my life.
Although I've had so many fears
Losing my baby has been my greatest strife.

It's a pain so deep inside
That it's not visible to the naked eye.
My pain and suffering I've learned to hide,
But it's so real, I sometimes want to die.

After months of discussing the events that lead to the autopsy, Isidro and I felt it was necessary to do something about it. We didn't want the doctors to do the same with other grieving parents. The mistake was not fair, and it was even worse that our doctor tried to hide the mistake by asking us to give permission for an act that had already been done. Kika knew of a malpractice attorney, so she gave us the number to contact him for a consultation. The attorney took our case because he thought it was unjust how we were treated.

The lawsuit and our decision to move on got us through the following months. We had concluded that we were not going to be birth parents, so we contemplated the possibility of adopting a child. It had been a year since our loss, and we were tired of feeling sad. I gathered information about the steps for adopting, and though Isidro wasn't fully convinced at first, to see me happy, he went along with the idea. We attended a few seminars, but based on everything we learned, we knew that two disabled individuals would never be allowed to become adoptive parents.

The costs for adopting in the United States were astronomical, and the chances of getting a baby were slim. We were required to be medically evaluated, and we knew that our disabilities would become an issue for the agencies. Still, we took the steps necessary to become adoptive parents. We soon became discouraged when obstacle after obstacle was presented from the different adoption agencies. Although I had never given up before, I was beaten. I suggested to Isidro that we go on a summer vacation to celebrate our anniversary and get away from everything for a while. We took a cruise, but instead of sightseeing, we kept looking at every baby or child whose path we crossed. We hired a taxi driver to give us a personalized tour. We saw little children in poverty, begging for money. My heart broke as I saw children no older than five years old working the streets to get money. Intellectually, we had come to terms that we wouldn't be parents, but emotionally, it was obvious we were far from accepting it.

CHAPTER 18

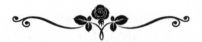

My parents were happy that we had gone on vacation. My mom was notably worried about me all the time. I had always been full of life, but I had lost that spark. For months she had tried to convince me that I was very blessed, pointing out all my blessings to me. She said, "You have a wonderful husband, a family that loves you, and a job you love. You are blessed and shouldn't ask for more." She knew me better, though; she knew that I would always want more and that I would always persist until I accomplished my goal.

The lawsuit against the doctor that delivered Cristian was still progressing. I didn't like to think much about it, but sometimes, the attorney would touch base to let us know what was going on. Because of the lawsuit, Isidro and I switched medical groups. Per my mom's and Father John's suggestion, I decided to transfer to a Catholic hospital. My mom was convinced that the doctor didn't do enough to save Cristian because he was viewed as a fetus and not a child. However, when I asked my attorney about this, the attorney assured me that Cristian was too premature and not viable for a court to rule malpractice. We switched to a group of doctors at Loyola University Hospital. I really liked our primary doctor and he suggested I go to a gynecologist for a yearly checkup.

Dreading this type of checkup, I had delayed the appointment until after my vacation. The doctor I saw was young, and we hit it off right away. He had been a student at Harper where I worked, so chatting about his experience there made the appointment go much smoother. I'd already transferred my medical records from Lutheran General Hospital, so he had my history. He didn't bring anything up, which I liked. He was very matter of fact and, from the beginning, I felt that my disability didn't matter to him. This is something I had never felt with my previous doctor.

My entire family suffered seeing me so devastated because of my previous losses. I know they would have done anything to help me. I started to spend more time with my little nieces and nephews. By now, I had twenty of them, from my side of the family alone. I even had a grandniece when one of Angelita's daughters, Veronica, had a baby girl. Our family was huge, but we all still managed to crowd into my mother's two-bedroom home for Christmas, Mother's Day, her birthday, and other holidays. The ones who lived furthest from her home were Reyna and me. On weekends, my mom had a revolving door. She was the conduit for us knowing what was going on in our family, so my brothers and sisters were aware of my struggles with adoption.

The cruise we took in July of 1999 gave me a glimpse of hope, though. I hadn't told Isidro at the time, but I started to wonder if we could become parents to a child in Mexico. I didn't even know if it was a possibility or what it would take, but I reserved that idea for me to pursue. Even my mom had noticed that I'd come back from vacation with a new attitude.

Kika agreed that looking for a child from Mexico would be a good idea if we wanted to be parents. Kika was married to Ernesto, who was from San Luis Potosí. Ernesto and Kika visited his family in San Luis often, so she said she would see what she could do to help me. One night on October 15, 1999, I got a call from a friend of Kika and Ernesto's who lived in Austin but was also originally from San Luis. She introduced herself and said, "Kika told me that you and your husband want to adopt a baby." I said, "Yes, we do." She then said, "I have a friend who is pregnant and due on November 20, and she wants to give her baby up for adoption." I couldn't believe what I was hearing. I told her to hold on and called Isidro to come near me. I said, "I am putting you on speakerphone so that Isidro can listen too." She said, "Are you interested in adopting the baby?" We both said yes at the same time.

We discussed the plan for getting our baby and agreed to travel to Mexico to pick him or her up and to pay all the birth expenses. I told her that I would consult with an adoption attorney so that everything would be ready by the time the baby was born. I immediately called Kika and verified that this call was legitimate. Kika confirmed that she had asked her friend to let her know if she knew of anyone wanting to give a child up for adoption. Kika gave her our number so that she could give us the good news.

Isidro and I were so happy, but at the same time, we were frightened to death. Could this be true? I was so scared of being disappointed, but for that night, I just wanted to be optimistic and happy. It was a Friday night, so we went out to celebrate and to make plans. We decided to take Monday off so that we could consult with an attorney. We also decided not to tell anyone, except my parents, until we were sure that this adoption would take place. It was another sleepless night, but this time, the night was full of anticipation and joy.

The week after that wonderful call, we made good headway in finding out information about the process for adoption. The attorney assured us that if the birth mom was willing to sign adoption papers, it would all be easy. She also explained how immigration worked in these cases. We hired the attorney and she agreed to draw the adoption papers so that they could be ready when the time came for us to go and get the baby. We were overjoyed with the good news. I also asked Harper's Human Resources Department how we could add the baby on my insurance plan. I made a list of everything that I needed to buy to welcome this new family member into our home.

On the following Friday, October 22, Kika's friend called us again. At first, I thought she was calling because she forgot to tell us some information or had some questions. She said, "Are you sitting down?" Again, I put her on speakerphone so that we could both listen. She said, "The baby came three weeks prematurely and was born earlier today." I said, "What? Are you sure?" Without hesitation, she responded, "Yes. I saw her, and she is so beautiful." I asked, "So it's a girl? Is she OK?" Quickly she said, "Oh yes. She was born healthy."

We sighed in relief because she was born without health issues. Afraid of her response, I then asked, "And we can still adopt her?" Isidro and I looked at each other waiting for her answer. She said, "Of course. That is why I am calling. When can you come to get her?" I told her that, since it was Friday, we probably couldn't fly out until the following week because we needed to notify our employers and we needed to meet with our lawyer. But we agreed to be in Mexico the following Friday. This would be a phone call I would never forget. Isidro and I stayed up late, making a list of all the things we had to do. There were a million things, but we were eager to make the trip and welcome our baby girl into our family.

On the Monday after the call, full of excitement, I talked to Tom at work about the adoption and my need to take some time off. I also emailed about half the college, letting them know that I was traveling to go pick up my baby. Luckily, I was approved for a leave because of the adoption. I of course let my departmental coworkers know, even though I felt bad because Bill had just started to work in disability services and now, I was taking off out of the blue. Some people assumed that the adoption had long been in the works and that I had kept it all a secret. They couldn't believe how fast everything had happened, and I told them I couldn't believe it either. I had so much to do. My list was long, and I hoped to get everything done prior to my departure that coming Friday.

I have always been blessed with good friends along the way. Another coworker and friend, Vicki, was so excited for me. She had a seven-year-old girl herself, and her daughter meant the world to her. She was very aware of my previous challenges in becoming a mother, so she was thrilled that this was happening to me. Unbeknownst to me, later that same day she heard my great news, she went to JCPenney and bought a bunch of pink baby items. I think she cleaned out the store. I am so grateful because I was not prepared to welcome a newborn and couldn't even begin to imagine everything that a new baby needed. Vicki purchased the cutest outfits, diapers, bottles, pacifiers, soft blankets, and many other thoughtful gifts. This generosity made one of the best times in my life so much less stressful so that I could just focus on my joy. Her generosity continued long after this; she shared with me many barely used items that her daughter no longer needed.

On Tuesday, we met with our lawyer. She informed us that they had not processed the immigration paperwork yet but that it was as simple as just taking the adoption papers to the embassy. I visited my parents to give them the news, and they couldn't believe it. I think my mom thought I had lost my marbles because she kept asking me if I was sure. She was of course also concerned about Isidro and me traveling on our own and wondered how we would be able to bring the newborn back. But my sister-in-law Irene had volunteered to go with us to help, and my brother-in-law Ernesto had volunteered to go as well, giving him a good excuse to go visit his parents. Isidro and I purchased the airplane tickets, but we decided to fly to Austin and then drive to San Luis in a rented minivan. We thought this would both be easier and would also give Isidro an opportunity to share the news with his parents.

Our angel from heaven was the most beautiful baby I had ever seen. She was so precious that I couldn't believe she was our baby. We were tired from our trip, so we rested in Kika's friend's house. I didn't want to be separated from my tiny baby, so she slept right by me. During the night, I would check to make sure she was breathing, reminding me of the stories my mom told me of when I was a baby and I slept on her lap. She was dressed in a beautiful pink outfit and wrapped in a simple flowered blanket. I noticed that she had a large silver charm attached to her outfit with a safety pin. I learned that her birth mother had attached the charm to her. I never met her, but I vowed to always thank her from afar. Our baby girl was as rosy as her outfit, though I did notice what seemed like a bruise by her upper lip. I bottle fed her a couple of times during the night, loving how she moved her little lips. I was feeling nauseous myself, wondering if it was just nerves and exhaustion.

The morning after I'd I held my daughter through the night for the very first time, we headed to get our paperwork in order so that we would all be able to travel back home together. Ernesto drove since he was most familiar with the area. We were told to go to the city hall in a small town called La Tapona in San Luis Potosí, which we could only get to by driving up several very narrow, winding dirt roads. We were going up a mountain and I just held my baby tight and avoided looking out the window. At one point, we had to stop for an older man passing with his horse. I also saw little children who were dressed in thin white dirty pants and shirts further up the road. I don't know what I was expecting, but when Ernesto told me we were there, I couldn't believe it. This city hall was a rugged wooden barn in the middle of nowhere. The wood appeared to be rotting—I could see right through the cracks of the planks. Irene held our baby as we went inside this "official" location.

There was another couple talking to a man behind a table who was typing on an old-fashioned typewriter. The couple held a baby, and I felt so bad when I heard the tiny infant coughing. They were registering the baby because the mother had given birth at her home. Isidro and I had already discussed girls' names just like we had for boys' names. When it was our turn, we registered our baby as Ariel Virginia Herrera. Her middle name was after the most important woman in my life, my mother. Ernesto and Irene were our witnesses. The typewriter made a loud click each time he turned the knob to answer the next question. It took slightly longer because of the barely functional typewriter. The worker gave us her birth certificate, and we left.

It was hard to believe that Ariel had been born in that destitute town. Yet again, I remembered that I was also born in a similar-looking town. I knew then that Ariel's birth mom had made the best decision, though likely a difficult one. On our way back, I prayed and thanked God for the little miracle in my hands, and I swore that I would give her the best life I could. I quietly said a prayer for Ariel's mom, thanking her for the sacrifice she made that had filled Isidro and me with such joy. I couldn't wait to get home to Chicago and start our life as a loving family.

Because the Day of the Dead and All Saints' Day are big holidays in Mexico, we had to wait a couple of days before traveling to Monterrey, where the US Embassy was located. We drove there and booked a hotel room so we could rest for the night before waking up to go to the embassy early the next day. We found out that Ariel had some lungs on her that night, though. A nervous wreck, I feared that all her loud crying meant something was wrong with her. I rocked her and gave her the formula. I was also instructed by Kika's friend to put some chamomile in her bottle, which I found odd. I couldn't wait to get home to have her checked by my doctor who was not only an internal medicine doctor but also a pediatrician.

Once everything was in order, we were able to head back home. The chamomile must have worked because Ariel was sound asleep when we crossed the border and didn't make a peep. I think that the agents weren't even aware that we had a newborn in our van. Ariel slept like a tiny angel, and I still couldn't believe that she was ours. I adored her from the moment we saw her. There was no doubt in my mind that I couldn't love her more even if she was my birth child. She already owned my heart and I would do anything to protect her. I was in awe of the miracle she was.

We briefly stopped at my in-law's house so they could meet Ariel. We were going to fly to Chicago the same day, November 3. Isidro's parents were so happy that their son now had a complete family. They were sad that we didn't stay longer but understood when I told them that my priority was to make sure that Ariel was well. I was neither sure of the circumstances of her birth nor why she was born prematurely nor what it meant for her health. I had already made an appointment for a checkup for the day after we arrived. At the same time, I wanted to be checked out because I was not feeling well either.

We decided to stop by my parents' house first before we went to our own home. Ariel had the same effect on my parents as she had had on me. I was pleasantly surprised that they immediately fell in love with her. It was surprising only because, when I was first thinking of adopting, my father had a conversation with me that made me think he might feel differently about an adopted grandchild. He'd said, "Are you sure you will love someone else's baby?" I'd said, "Of course." He'd said, "We cannot force to feel love for anyone." I'd been a bit offended and said, "So are you saying that you won't love an adopted grand-child?" He'd looked at me and said, "To be honest, I don't know. But I do hope so because I want to love what you love." As I saw him look at Ariel that day, though, I was certain that if I asked him the same question again, he would quickly respond with a yes. Though it had been a difficult conversation, I think it helped me to be one hundred percent sure of my decision to adopt. I loved my baby girl!

On the second day Ariel was in the United States, she had her first checkup. Our doctor was expecting us and checked her from head to toe. He was surprised about the chamomile and said that she didn't need it. He changed her formula and told me that every-thing looked good. Furthermore, the mark I saw on her lip was a birthmark that he thought would disappear as she got older. Her weight and height were good for being almost two weeks old. I was so happy that she was healthy and that I didn't have to worry about any health concerns.

My doctor then examined me and confirmed what I feared. He did a pregnancy test and it came out positive. I was pregnant again and expecting a child. He gave me a referral to go see the same doctor that I had seen for a gynecology exam. I don't know what I felt. All the trauma of my past pregnancies rushed to my mind. Would I be able to go through this again? As I started to panic, I looked at Ariel who was kicking wildly. I told myself, *Don't worry. You already have an angel.* I repeated that thought over and over until I calmed down. I knew that Ariel would be my strength to withstand anything that came to me.

I went to see Dr. Sean, my ob-gyn doctor. I left Ariel with my mom, who had convinced me to stay at her house at least for a couple of weeks until I got used to caring for a newborn. I was happy she asked because I was nervous about not knowing what to do if she got sick. After my exam, Dr. Sean congratulated me and when I told him I had just adopted a child, instead of being in shock as I expected, he gave me a high five. I was expecting him to feel sorry for me or wonder how dare I think I could handle two babies. But this again confirmed that he saw me as a fully accomplished woman who just happened to have a disability. He even joked and said, "Too much of that wine-and-dine celebrating your adoption, eh?" In all seriousness, he said, "I don't see your pregnancy as high risk. What I see as high risk is your nervousness." I told him that my previous doctor had said that my body wasn't made for babies. He said, "Well, good thing you changed doctors. Maybe his body isn't made for babies, but your body is." For my own peace of mind, he recommended that I take a longer leave from work than the six weeks I was planning to take. His reassurance and my precious angel are what would help me through my fourth pregnancy.

Harper College offered wonderful benefits for faculty. I was approved for a medical leave because of the possible complications with my pregnancy. After using all my sick days, I qualified to go onto short term disability, so I received sixty percent of my salary. I also made the decision to use my wheelchair regularly. First, I found that I was able to handle Ariel better than when I used crutches. Second, I was concerned about falls and possibly injuring Ariel or my pregnancy. I was still cautiously optimistic, preparing myself for a repetition of what had happened in the past.

After a couple of weeks, Isidro, Ariel, and I went back to our condo. Isidro went back to work while I took care of Ariel at home. I had to figure out a way to safely transport her to other rooms since I had a difficult time carrying her while still pushing my wheelchair. So, I took a rolling basket that I used when I did laundry and lined it with puffy blankets, then laid Ariel in it. I could pull the cart as I pushed myself. At first, I was so scared of something happening to her, but after a few weeks, I learned that I was creative and was perfectly able to care for her on my own. When I cooked dinner, I would roll her over so I could always see her. Although we purchased a crib for her, I found that the cart was more manageable, since I struggled to put her inside the crib from a sitting-down position. She ended up sleeping with us for easy access during the night.

Ariel was a fussy little baby. She didn't sleep well at night. I would sit and rock her and sometimes I would fall asleep while she was still wide awake. I tried all the suggestions that were given to me from my family and friends. Isidro and I figured out that when she was in our car, she slept the whole ride. Several times, after being desperate to get her to sleep, we would load into our car and go for a midnight ride. During the day, she would take long naps, and though I tried to sleep then as well, I just was not able to sleep during the daytime. I was often bored, so I called Tom to ask if I could do anything to help the department. So, during my leave, I created our policy manual. I'd write parts and then have him review them. This made time go a bit quicker.

My desire was for Ariel to become a United States citizen. I decided to also put my time toward filing the application on my own, although some people thought it would be best to hire an immigration attorney. But my year of law school had given me the confidence to believe that I could apply on my own. I wanted a head start because I knew it would take longer than a year. When Ariel was barely a couple of months old, Isidro and I took her to Walgreens to take a passport picture. I was sure that Ariel was the youngest person ever to take a picture at that Walgreens. The young man looked panicked but was able to lay her on her blanket on the floor to take the picture. Once I sent the completed application, I just waited for a court date.

When Ariel was three months old, I asked Father John if he would baptize her. I got permission from the parish we were attending in Palatine for Father John to perform this important sacrament. I asked my brother Lalo and my sister-in-law Irene to be the godparents.

Isidro and I made this decision because we were extremely grateful that Irene had volunteered to go to Mexico to assist us when we adopted Ariel. We believed that if something were to happen to us, Ariel would be well taken care of by them. Irene bought Ariel the most precious white dress. She looked like an absolute angel. My mother attended the ceremony along with some family and friends. I chose to stand for some of the pictures although I was using my wheelchair almost entirely now.

We were so blessed to have found a wonderful group of doctors and nurses. They were so helpful. Whenever Ariel got sick or went for her vaccinations and well-baby appointments, I could call the clinic to let them know we'd arrived, and then one of the nurses would come outside, grab Ariel, and take her in. This was extremely helpful, especially during the winter months when it would take us too long to get her in safely. Ariel, for the most part, was a healthy baby. She did struggle with ear infections and sometimes with a bit of asthma. She was very sensitive to loud noises and would get easily startled. We were really getting attached spending the entire day together. I loved her more than I ever imagined.

My pregnancy was going well. Ironically the projected due date was on my birthday, May 17. I sometimes honestly forgot that I was even pregnant because I was constantly busy with Ariel. Everything took more time. Bathing Ariel took me a couple of hours. Between changing her diaper, feeding her, and bathing, my entire day was consumed. I told myself that I wouldn't get excited until my third trimester, or week twenty-four. On the other hand, I loved my baby the minute I knew I was pregnant. Because I was always sitting, I hoped that the baby wouldn't be affected. Dr. Sean did periodic ultrasounds and he always said the baby was fine. This time, I did want to know the gender of the baby and found out it was a girl. I started to daydream of how wonderful it would be to have two little girls so close in age. We started to think of names once we got to the second trimester. In choosing the name, Isidro and I wanted to make sure that the name could be pronounced both in English and Spanish.

Ever since I could remember, I had a fascination with angels. Most people thought that I chose Ariel's name based on *The Little Mermaid*, when in fact I chose it because of the Archangel Ariel who was the Angel of Nature. After much thought and discussion, we ended up with three possible names that we liked for the baby I was expecting: Crystal, Julieta, and Ariana. In researching the names, we decided on Ariana because it derived and meant "Oh Holy One," in Greek. Plus, just like Ariel, it would be easy to pronounce. And as a bonus, both names began with the same three letters. Of course, we never contemplated the tongue twister it would be when we tried to get both of their attention in a hurry.

Because I was always sitting, I didn't begin showing until later in the pregnancy. I was so grateful when we reached the seven months of pregnancy. Everything that I read indicated that there was a great survival rate for babies born after the seventh month of pregnancy. Because Ariel was still so little, we didn't venture out much, especially during the winter. However, once we crossed my seventh month of pregnancy, we were able to go out to dinner. It was the first time that we'd gone out as a family, other than to the doctor or my parents' home. I immediately noticed the stares of people. I was sure that they were being judgmental and thinking, *Where is the baby's mother? I can't believe they let two disabled people go out with such a little baby.* I had learned to build a thick shell and not care what people may or may not be thinking. However, I started to notice that Isidro had a totally different view on disability.

Perhaps because the onset of our disability was at a different age, we saw disability through a different lens. I contracted polio as an infant, so being disabled was all I knew. Not to mention, I was an educator, so I saw an opportunity to teach others about disabilities instead of getting irritated and responding in a defensive way. Yet Isidro didn't get juvenile rheumatoid arthritis until much later. He had experienced life without a disability. He was now unable to do things that he remembered he could do. For example, he always liked music and had started to learn to play the guitar, yet now he couldn't hold it due to the position of his arms and the lack of range of motion. So, it wasn't surprising that he would be bothered by the stares more often.

Isidro and I would be millionaires if we had a dollar for each time someone commented about our disabilities. Frequently, complete strangers asked us, "What happened to you?" Or, "Were you in an accident?" Immediately, I would put on my educator hat and want to give an explanation such as, "I have polio and my husband has arthritis." I did this until Isidro pointed out something I hadn't contemplated. He said, "Cuali, why do you tell them our personal information when they don't even know our names?" That question was so spot on. Why should anyone know my disability before they knew my name? Wasn't I fighting my entire life wanting to be known as a person and not my label? From then on, I changed my approach and when I was asked about my disability, I would teach them that the first question they should ask is, "What is your name?"

I was thirty-five years old and was accustomed to people making invasive remarks or ignoring me as if I didn't even exist. When I was still single, I often took many of my nieces and nephews out to various locations, and there were times when we went to a store and a notably younger niece or nephew would be asked, "What color does she want?" Or they would even say something as overt as, "Tell her the coupon she is using is expired." It was so obvious that, to them, I was nonexistent, or, in the best-case scenario, my intelligence was being questioned. I could probably write a whole separate book about the multitude of examples I have of times when others would dismiss me because they preferred to communicate with a child rather than to try to interact with me. The many microaggressions I encountered then, though, didn't even begin to prepare me for the experiences I would face as a disabled, expectant mother.

Buying maternity clothes when I began showing was more than challenging. Some stores would assume that I was looking in the wrong department and would say, "If you are looking for plus-sized clothes, it is to your right." Sometimes the clerks would say the rudest comments to me, without realizing they were offensive. For example, once I wanted to buy a blouse and, trying to be nice, the cashier said, "Do you need a gift receipt? Whoever is getting this will surely like it." It's as if women in wheelchairs could not possibly be pregnant! Little did they know, I had been pregnant four times.

But, just as there are ignorant individuals, there are also many wonderful, compassionate people. Ariel had her six-month well-baby appointment, and as usual, I called from my car and asked if someone could come out to help me bring Ariel in. My primary doctor and the nurses were fully aware of my pregnancy, so they were especially sensitive to my need for assistance. One of the nurses came out and said, "Today we are going to use a different examining room than the one with the low table."

As I transferred into my wheelchair, I said, "That's fine, Ariel is the one getting examined." We went inside and the nurse led me to a different room, which was the one farthest down. When she opened the door, I saw streamers hanging, balloons tied to the chairs, a small cake on the doctor's desk, and gifts on the bed. Confused, I asked, "Should we use another room? Looks like you will be having a party." She giggled and said, "Don't be silly; it's for you." I couldn't believe it and began to tear up. She said, "Everyone here wanted to throw you a little baby shower." I was speechless, and between sniffles, all I could say was, "Thank you; thank you so much." The goodness of people never ceases to amaze me.

The help from the clinic and their niceness was so appreciated. Though I didn't think I was showing, I did notice that I was having a difficult time getting around, especially caring for Ariel now that she was bigger and heavier. On bad days, I started to wonder if I had been irresponsible in not listening to God's clear message that I shouldn't be a mother. I would start to feel sorry for myself and become overwhelmed, not knowing what I would do with *two* little babies. I wondered if I had gotten myself into a situation that was too much for me to handle. I think the hormones were acting up because so many doubts clouded my mind.

Another constant fear I had went back to the question my dad had once asked me. I knew that I loved Ariel with all my heart but wondered whether this would change after giving birth. Or, equally as bad, what if I didn't love her as much as I love Ariel? I didn't share these doubts with anyone, but it was affecting me to the point where I was almost unable to function. I was exhausted all the time. I tried to keep up with keeping the house tidy, doing laundry, cooking, and caring for a high-maintenance six-month-old. I even wondered if I was doing something wrong because Ariel was so clingy and sensitive to so many things. All I could do was pray and ask for God's strength.

It was always amazing how my mom knew me better than anyone. She saw my struggles and knew that I would push through no matter what. One weekend when we went to visit, she said, "Cauli, why don't you come and live here so I can help you?" I waited a second, just a second, and then said, "I thought you would never ask." I started to cry and told her all my fears and how I was so tired. My mom wasn't the type that would support with pity, though. She would demand strength and would always offer food to make things better. As I started to cry, she said, "Come, and I will fry you an egg."

Isidro and I decided to take up my mother on her offer, so we moved in with my parents and used the back rooms as we had done before. We also started to wonder how we would handle going back to work. My mom was willing to care for the girls, but how would we bring them to her all the way from Palatine, which was about twenty-five miles away? We concluded that we had to sell our condo and look for a house that was close to my mother so she could watch our girls. I loved our home, so it was a difficult decision. However, as parents we were willing to do anything for the benefit of our daughters.

We used the same realtor we'd used when we first bought our condo. We had maintained it in excellent condition, so it was on the market for only one day before we received an offer. We had lived in it for close to four years, and we sold it for twenty thousand dollars more than what we bought it for. I was three weeks from my due date, and I had to pack and care for Ariel simultaneously. But I have always been so supported by my family. My mom helped tremendously, as did my brothers and sisters and nieces and nephews.

As we prepared to move, we were planning to keep some of our furniture for a future home, but the buyers of the condo loved our décor so much that they made an offer to buy the house furnished. Since we would have had to rent storage space anyway, we took the offer. I had many very happy moments in the first home we owned, and I just prayed we would continue to be blessed in the same way.

CHAPTER 19

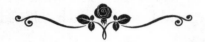

Living back home brought me peace. I knew that I would be well protected because no one knew me better than my mom. With her, it was OK to be scared and worried. I could put my guard down and not feel like I was always having to prove myself to others. I welcomed her help and knew that she would be stern when needed. I was getting so anxious because my due date was around the corner. I started seeing Dr. Sean every week, and he was constantly monitoring how my pregnancy was progressing.

A week before my due date, I woke up and the world was spinning. I had severe vertigo, and the dizziness made me nauseous. I was overtaken by the fear that something was wrong and was almost having a nervous breakdown, crying without any consolation. My mom asked, "Do you have sharp pain?" I would close my eyes tight and say, "No, everything is just spinning." My mom always thought that food was the remedy for any malady. She went to the kitchen and brought me a freshly made arroz con leche (rice pudding). I said, "If I eat anything, I will throw up." She looked at Isidro and said, "Maybe ask the doctor what we can do?" Isidro called Dr. Sean's office and left a message for the nurse. The nurse immediately called back and directed Isidro to take me to Loyola Hospital's emergency room. My mother called Rique, who lived across the street, to come help me get into the car.

The attending doctor examined me to determine if my vertigo was attributed to being in labor. He asked many questions to understand all my symptoms. He said, "Your symptoms don't seem to be related to your pregnancy. You are not in labor." Both Isidro and I were puzzled. If I wasn't about to give birth, then what was wrong with me? The doctor continued and said, "I will call your doctor and order an ultrasound to make sure all is well with the baby." After he left the room, Isidro asked, "Are you still dizzy?" I replied, "Everything is spinning. Everything is rotating to the right." I had never felt anything like this, and I was overly anxious. I thought to myself, *What if this spinning never stops?*

After my ultrasound, Dr. Sean said, "She is not quite ready to come into the world." I asked, "What's wrong with me then?" He said, "You've lost your marble." I knew he was joking, but frankly, I wasn't in the mood for it. He must have noticed my expression because he then said, "In all seriousness, you have a condition called Benign Paroxysmal Positional Vertigo, or BPPV for short." He explained that it was triggered by an inner ear infection that causes the dizziness. He said, "I said you lost your marble because a little crystal in the ear came loose and it causes the world to spin." He showed me how to do some exercises that would send the "marble" back into the right place inside my ear. I thought to myself, *Leave it to me to get the oddest type of condition.*

The doctor discharged me and said that, although there was medication for the vertigo, he would prefer that I just do the exercises. He reassured me that the condition was not serious and that I would be back to normal within a couple of days. He said, "Don't drive, either, because they will think you are drunk." I was so relieved to know that my little one was fine and just too comfortable to want to enter the world. At home I followed the doctor's instructions and did the exercise every thirty minutes. I was determined to get the marble back in its socket.

My birthday came and went with no sign of Ariana wanting to join our family yet. I went for my weekly checkup and asked Dr. Sean, "Why is there a delay in her birth?" He said, "The due date is an estimate; it's likely we had the wrong date." He also said that, as a precaution, he recommended a C-section because of the curvature of my spine. He'd been mentioning this throughout the pregnancy but wanted to wait to see how I progressed before making a definite decision. But when he saw my desperation, he said, "I will schedule the C-section for either Wednesday, June 7, 2000, or June 8, 2000. What do you prefer?" I barely let him finish when I quickly responded, "June 7." Jokingly he said, "Is seven your lucky number?" I said, "No, it just comes before eight and I want her out!"

In addition to helping me watch Ariel, my mother was busy with her garden. Every year she would convert her yard into a glorious paradise with her many flowers. Her favorite outing was to go to any store where they sold dirt. My dad even said that he had once started to count how many flowerpots she had but had gotten tired by the time he reached at least a hundred. She didn't hide her love for her garden and took pride in showing off her creations to anyone who came to visit. My mom had this amazing touch that would make anything grow and flourish. I didn't inherit those traits at all. If anyone ever gave me any plants, I would show mercy to them by giving them to my mother. I even made a cactus die once. During this tough time of my pregnancy, I found it relaxing to sit outside on a blanket with Ariel, watching her play as my mom gardened.

On Monday, two days before the C-section was scheduled, I received a call from Dr. Sean. He sounded horrible, coughing and with a hoarse voice. He said, "I am sorry, but I have a terrible bug. I will not be able to do the C-section on Wednesday." I said, "Oh no. Sorry you are sick, but what will I do?" He coughed, cleared his throat, and said, "Well, we can reschedule it for the following Wednesday, or if you don't want to change, one of my partners can do the C-section." Without hesitation, I said, "Let your partner do it." He said, "OK, thank you for your understanding. I am sorry I won't be there to welcome Ariana." I hung up the phone, and for a minute I felt guilty for not rescheduling. However, I also knew that another week would be too long to wait. But I was disappointed that Dr. Sean wouldn't be there for my baby's birth.

The day finally arrived. We were instructed to get to the hospital by 7 AM. I was as nervous as I'd been on the flight to go get Ariel. As I was being prepared for the procedure, I almost had a panic attack. The memory of that awful day when I had to part from my son, whom I loved so much, crept to my mind and wouldn't let me relax. I was wheeled into the operating room at around 9 AM. Dr. Sean's partner was a woman doctor whom I had met once. She briefly introduced herself and said all would be well.

Ariana Angelina Herrera was welcomed to the world on June 7, 2000, at 10:40 AM at Loyola Hospital in Maywood, Illinois. Her middle name was after her paternal grandmother, Isidro's mom. She was so tiny, weighing only six pounds, four ounces and measuring nineteen inches. She was this beautiful masterpiece that couldn't have been more precious. I held her in my arms when I awoke from the anesthesia. This type of surgery I didn't mind. I was so full of emotion that I couldn't help but cry. I told myself, *I did it! She is here, she is alive, she is beautiful, and she is perfectly healthy.* I couldn't thank God enough. Isidro and I hugged as I said, "My body *was* made for babies." He knew exactly what I was referring to.

My mom and my niece Estela came to the hospital. I was in a lot of pain and full of anxiety, but still very happy. I kept checking her little hands, to make sure she was completely whole. Memories of Cristian's undeveloped body came to me as I contemplated the miracle in my arms. My mom held her, and her love was pouring out of her heart. She didn't find one single defect on her new grandchild. I couldn't believe how this little being had just completed my perfect family. I couldn't understand how I had been able to live without her.

The day after Ariana was born, my mom came to visit us again. She had left Ariel with my sister Tere and my brother-in-law, Ismael. She sat by my bed and while holding Ariana, she said, "You know, I keep asking for extensions." I said, "What do you mean?" Without taking her eyes off Ariana, she said, "Since you had polio, I have been asking God for extensions." Again, I asked, "What do you mean?" She replied, "First, when I was getting my kidney removed, I asked

God for life so that I could take care of you." She continued, "Then I asked God for enough life to see you stand." Still holding Ariana lovingly, she said, "Then I wanted more life to see you successful." I was now getting her point and asked, "Then what?" "Then I asked for life to see you settled with someone who could love you." She took a deep sigh, and said, "And He has given me life to see you accomplish all of this." She smiled and looked at me and said, "So now, I will need to start asking God for an extension so that I can help you raise your beautiful daughters. Yes, I will do that." My heart filled with even more admiration for the wonderful woman who gave me life twice.

My discharge was two days after my C-section. I couldn't wait to go home to my little Ariel. I was in so much pain because I used my abdomen muscles to move. I felt as if a truck had run over me. Ariana had been brought to me so I could get her ready. She was so much smaller than Ariel. She made these tiny moans and I wondered if something was wrong. I couldn't stop looking at her. I moved slowly to get myself dressed and then transferred into my wheelchair. I picked her up and put her on the bed to dress her with the little outfit that I had selected. I had not done a good job in my selection because two Arianas could have fit in that one outfit.

Isidro and my mom came in as I was dressing her. He sat down and said, "Can I hold her?" I smiled and said, "She is yours too." I then asked, "How is Ariel?" He told me that my nieces were having fun with her. My sister Tere had taken her across the street to her house so that my mom could come to the hospital. The nurse came with her discharge papers. I asked my mom to grab Ariana so that we could go. She put her on the bed and swaddled her with the blanket. Isidro left to get the car while we went down to the bottom level.

What a welcome Ariana and I received! A huge stork was on the front lawn with a sign saying WELCOME ARIANA, JUNE 7, 2000. My niece Velia had ordered it as a surprise. My sister was keeping an eye out from her home. When she saw that we had arrived, Tere and Ismael came over with Ariel. Ariel began dancing, eagerly wanting me to hold her. My poor baby, it was the first time I had been separated from her.

Boy, did she look big! I couldn't believe how grown up she looked compared to Ariana when Ariel was only seven and half months older. I closed my eyes for a second and thanked God for my blessings which were all around me. For sure, life was not always a valley of tears.

Everyone came to meet the new addition to the family. Ariana became my parents' twenty-second grandchild. We had to get creative settling into my parents' tiny home. I only had twelve weeks left before having to return to work. Ariana would only be three months and Ariel would be almost a year. So, I made the difficult decision to not breastfeed Ariana. It would be too difficult with my working twenty miles away. I also felt that I wanted to treat both girls the same and feared that the closeness I would have when feeding Ariana wouldn't be fair to Ariel.

My love for them was the same for both. All my fears disappeared as soon as I had them both and realized that I would give my life for either of them. I also loved seeing how my parents and the rest of the family treated Ariel with the same love as Ariana. This convinced me that love is what unites us, not that I had given birth to one child and adopted the other.

I felt blessed, and my faith became stronger, realizing that God always has a divine plan. Perhaps I had to go through the difficult pain of two miscarriages and a premature birth so that I would be ready to adopt Ariel, who needed loving parents to raise her. Losing Cristian stopped being as painful because I felt that God had rewarded me for all my suffering. I couldn't imagine my life without either of my two beautiful daughters.

It was not easy for me to have two infants or, as some people referred to them, Irish twins. The first couple of months were particularly difficult because my mobility was gravely affected because of the pain caused by my C-section. I had difficulty even caring for myself. I remember vividly how my sister Angelita had to come into the bathroom after I had showered to help me dress. My tears just fell as I acknowledged my limitations and accepted such intimate help. I realized then that moving back with my mom had been the best decision. My mom became my girls' second mom, and both would grow to rightfully call her Mama China.

Although I had thought that I'd started using my wheelchair for the safety of Ariel and my pregnancy, I soon realized that I wasn't able to walk anymore. I put on my brace and attempted to walk, but my spine had become even more curved and I felt very unsure of myself. My mom wanted one last picture of me standing. So, we went out to her garden, and Isidro and I carried one child each, Isidro with Ariel, and me with Ariana. It was a difficult picture to take because, deep down, I knew that I wouldn't ever stand again. That image of the girls dressed as twins in blue striped short sets will remain etched in my memory until the day I die.

Caring for two babies is difficult for anyone, but it's even more difficult when both parents have disabilities. I would sit in the middle of the bed with one baby on each side of me as I fed them their bottles. Ariana was a calm baby, which I appreciated since Ariel demanded so much more attention. Some weeks were especially difficult because, if one got sick, the other would soon follow. The doctor and nurses continued to be so supportive with helping me bring them in, especially now that I had two little ones. I think they either felt sorry for me or admired me for getting into this situation and pushing through like a champ. Knowing them, it was most likely the latter.

Returning to work was both stressful and a relief. I had been out for almost an entire year, from October 1999 to September 2000. It was stressful to figure out a good balance, especially because, after work, I would be going to my second "job" to relieve my mother. It was also a relief, though, because for close to twelve months, I had been focusing on my girls one hundred percent of the time. I was now able to focus on other things and, at least during my commute, have some alone time. I also had the advantage of not worrying about them, knowing they were in good hands. If they were ill with a bug, I would jokingly tell my mom, "Please get them well by the time I get home." I had full trust in my mom. I never had to miss work unless I had to take them to the doctor, and even then, Isidro and I took turns.

Getting reacclimated took time because of how rapidly things change in academia, but working with students with disabilities was still my fascination. I returned with new ideas and began taking more leadership roles. I became the coordinator of the learning services, with the responsibility for hiring, training, and supervising adjunct Learning Disability Specialists. Tom trusted my ability and knew that I would work very hard. I always maintained my own load of students because it was clearly what I enjoyed most. We had a great team, and we cared for each other. We were always willing to try new things for the benefit of students. We regularly engaged in professional development opportunities by attending conferences and taking classes. I was tenured for the second time shortly before going on maternity leave, so not needing to worry about tenure any longer definitely helped me be more confident.

Our department had a long history of service to students who are deaf and who benefited from various grants to better support them. As I previously mentioned earlier, to better support deaf culture on campus, we decided to change the name of our department from the Center for Students with Disabilities (CSD) to Access and Disability Services (ADS). I had started to think about disability as a culture and began to realize that my disability wasn't what was bad. Rather, I began to understand that lack of access and people's attitudes toward disabilities were really what affected me. I think this is when I stopped believing that being in a wheelchair was negative.

I was now using the wheelchair all the time. Because Harper is a big campus, it made sense for me to use it permanently. To transport my wheelchair, I was still using the apparatus on top of my car. This was a very useful tool that gave me independence. However, during the winter, it was less than reliable. It would sometimes stop functioning because of the cold or the snow. On top of that, pushing my manual wheelchair in snow was extremely difficult, especially when I had the girls with me. As time went on, I found myself struggling to push up ramps or far distances. My arms began to feel sore. I knew that I would soon have to figure out an alternative.

Being a wheelchair user with two little girls required a lot of creativity. In addition to a double stroller, I would also use the kind of pouch people usually put on their backs to carry a baby. Instead I would put it on my chest facing forward and put one of the girls in there while I pushed the other one in a lighter stroller. I found the perfect bassinet on wheels for home, which I used to bring the girls from room to room. Raising two babies so close in age was fun but also a lot of work. When one was calm, the other would be cranky. When one was sleeping, the other would be wide awake. They couldn't be more different. They became our lives when we were not at work.

Our first public celebration for our full family of four was my parents' fiftieth wedding anniversary in September 2000. Ariel was almost a year, and Ariana was three months old. This was a celebration we couldn't miss. The Mass was at the church where I got married, and Father Luis, one of my friends from DePaul, celebrated the Mass. The reception was close to our home, which meant it would be easy for us to leave if the girls became uncooperative. It was a lively party, and I loved seeing my parents so happy. My mom was already sixty-seven and my dad was seventy-five. All my brothers and sisters sang my parents' favorite song, "Renunciacion." All the poverty and suffering the family had overcome was erased with our happiness that day.

As the girls began to grow, Isidro and I began to have discussions about how we wanted them to live full lives. We didn't want our disabilities to impact their opportunities. We wondered if some day they would resent having to live with two people who were so challenged. We tried not to worry too much and decided to just do the best we could by always showing them our love. At the very least, I was sure that they couldn't be part of a better family. They were surrounded by their grandparents, aunts, uncles, and a bunch of cousins. My nieces were always willing to come over to help with them. Olivia and Vanessa, Angelita's daughters, would come over to help with bath time any time they could.

We baptized Ariana when she was almost four months old. We chose Rique and his wife Betty to be her godparents. Rique and I had always been close, and I knew he would do all he could to make sure Ariana would be safe in my absence. Besides, Rique's daughter Jenny was also watched by my parents, so I knew they would grow up like sisters. Father John, once again, gave her the sacrament of baptism in a beautiful, intimate ceremony. I was content that Isidro and I were raising them as Catholics and that they would learn about Jesus. My faith had always carried me through the darkest times, so I wanted to make sure they inherited that from me.

We raised our girls, probably breaking a lot of the rules written in books about child safety. I read about the importance of child proofing a home, but as I read the suggested steps, I realized that none of those things would work for us. For example, one suggestion was to store bleach, soap, or other dangerous substances up high. Well, I couldn't access them if they were up high, so that wasn't an option. I would joke that my girls were raised among sharp objects and dangerous chemicals. But they were so smart that they knew those items were off limits for them. Similarly, for the sake of access, I couldn't use the recommended baby products. Small bathtubs wouldn't work because I couldn't bend down to them from my chair. Bending down to the actual bathtub wouldn't be safe for them either because then I couldn't hold them. So, my girls learned that the kitchen sink was a fun baby bathtub.

I was living the typical middle-class life, raising my girls while working. On weekends, we dedicated our time to grocery shopping, doing laundry, and spending time resting with the girls. My mom's house continued to be a revolving door where all my siblings would visit at least once during the weekend, which was a benefit I hadn't fully appreciated when we first decided to move into the back room at my parents' home. But I loved that my daughters were growing up so close to the family. My sister Tere and her husband Ismael would often ask if they could take Ariel to their house so that I could get some relief and just focus on Ariana. Tere was the first one to see Ariel walk. Tere and Ismael both had so much fun with her.

When Ariel was about a year and a half old, we finally received a notice for a hearing for her naturalization as a United States citizen. The appointment was going to be in front of a judge who would review the application and ask questions. We were nervous, and I began to wonder whether I should have hired an attorney after all. I prepared for the hearing, gathering documents and pictures, and writing down the sequence of events pertaining to her adoption. Isidro and I thought it would be best for him to remain at home with Ariel and Ariana so that I could go to court on my own. One of my nieces, Olivia, accompanied me downtown.

When we arrived at the courthouse, we went to the location of the hearing and were asked to wait. I was visibly nervous but couldn't help but compare it to the location where I had first gone to register Ariel. What a difference between this courthouse and the city hall in La Tapona. I had my binder ready, and, in my head, I ran through all the responses I had rehearsed for possible questions. They called Ariel's name, so I rolled into the judge's chamber. The judge was African American, and she was sitting behind her desk. On the side I noticed a bulletin board with pictures of little Asian-looking girls. As she was reviewing the application, I asked, "Are those girls your daughters?" She looked up, smiled, and said, "Yes, they are. Thank you; you are the first person who has contemplated the possibility of them being my girls." She cleared her throat and continued reviewing the application I had completed the year before. She then said, "Everything seems to be in order. Congratulations. Ariel is a US citizen." I couldn't believe it. She didn't even ask a question. I had been so nervous, but it was as if an angel had put his hand on her mouth so no questions would come out.

This merited a huge celebration. I decided to throw a party to celebrate Ariel's citizenship that would also be a surprise birthday party for Isidro. I rented a pizzeria and invited my whole family and a bunch of my friends. Since Isidro's family was in Texas, I asked his oldest sister to take videos of his family sending their birthday wishes. It was a wonderful celebration, and now Ariel would have the same benefits as if she had been born in the US. I was so thankful and proud that my whole family had citizenship in this country now.

Our little family of four was on a roll with celebrations. We also had to celebrate Ariana's first birthday! Rique and Betty offered their yard for the party, which was very convenient since they lived across the street, next to Tere's house. We bought a pinata that was bigger than Ariana. Ariana was very tiny but oh so smart. She was already walking by her birthday and had already proven herself to be an introvert. She didn't like big crowds and could entertain herself by herself with just about anything. We very quickly discovered that hiring a clown had not been a smart idea. Even though the adults loved him, Ariana wasn't too happy to be near him and Ariel wasn't terribly keen on him either.

Beyond these celebrations, though, the lawsuit against the doctor at Lutheran General Hospital was still pending. I was ready to put it behind me. They scheduled a deposition but because I had two babies, the lawyers agreed to do it at my mom's house. Several fancily dressed lawyers, along with a court reporter, set up around my kitchen table. Both attorneys asked questions, but my lawyer would chime in to let me know if I should respond or not. I was honest and expressed that I felt my son had been treated as tissue and not as a human being. I stressed that what was more disappointing was that the doctor had attempted to hide the mistake. The whole deposition lasted a couple of hours since Isidro also had to respond to questions.

Several weeks after the deposition, my lawyer called and asked if I'd consider a settlement if they made an offer. I reminded the lawyer that I commenced this case not for the money but because I didn't want other families to go through what I had. He asked, "What do you really want?" I responded, "I would like to get an apology from the doctor and a hospital policy made that no autopsies will be done without parental consent." He said, "OK, I will be in touch." Later the same week, my lawyer called again and said, "We have a trial date in two weeks."

Again, I went to the courthouse. I hoped that the trial wouldn't last long because I was missing days of work. I hated to miss work because my schedule was always full. Isidro went through security and up the elevator to the assigned court room. Our lawyer was already there. He was not the most personable person, but I had gotten to know his style and really came to respect him and his intelligence. We briefly greeted each other, and he directed us to where Isidro could sit on a bench and wait. A few minutes later he came out and said, "They made an offer. They agree to your terms of writing a letter of apology and changing the hospital policy, along with a payment of $50,000. Do you accept, or do you still want your day in court?" I looked at Isidro and then asked the lawyer, "What do you recommend?" He said, "You are getting what you wanted, and I don't guarantee you will get anything better." Isidro and I both wanted this over so that we could start fresh with our family. We accepted the settlement. After paying the attorneys, we ended up with about $29,000, the letter, and a confirmation of the hospital agreement for a policy change. We split the money and opened college funds for each of the girls, calling it the Cristian fund. We smiled when we said, "Someday we can tell the girls that their older brother sent them to college."

Isidro and I were relieved that these worries were now behind us. We wanted to focus on our family. We were home most of the time; going out with both girls was a challenge because they demanded a lot from us physically. After it became too difficult to buckle them into their car seats, we purchased a minivan for the extra space. I was able to get into the minivan by using a small portable stool to step up, and then Isidro could lift my wheelchair into the back. We always seemed to find a solution that allowed us to be active.

As a married couple, we knew we had a lot of blessings. We had a roof over our heads, good jobs, our beautiful daughters, each other, and a wonderful extended family. We were blessed that our family had been guarded from loss, besides Cristian, since Mama Petra died in 1988. In October 2001, shortly after Ariel turned two, Ismael, Tere's husband, was hospitalized with an unexpected diagnosis of cancer. Sadly, the surgery to remove his cancerous tumor was unsuccessful, which caused him to pass away a few days later. This shocked the family to the core. It was so difficult to see my sister Tere and her three kids so devastated. I didn't have the words to console my two nieces, Velia and Estela, who had traveled and spent so much time with me when I most needed it. Ismael also left a twelve-year-old son, Ismaelito, who would have to grow up during the toughest years of adolescence without him. The entire family cried for such a difficult loss. I was always going to have fond memories of a man who, though quiet and reserved, exuded love for his family and for my daughter Ariel. His bright smile would live in our memories long after he left this world.

CHAPTER 20

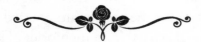

United as a family, we continued our life, even when a loved one had left our family. We were comfortable living in the back of my mom's house, but we were tight on space between the four of us, especially with the girls growing and needing more stuff. It was hard to believe we had been living in my mom's house for over a year. Isidro and I had known that the move would be temporary and that, eventually, we would want to have our own home again. Now that the school year was over and Ariel and Ariana were both over a year old and walking, we figured that the summer was a good time to look for a new place to live. We wanted to remain close to my mom for the girls' sake, even though it made for a longer commute to work for us both.

Even if we lived close, though, we were still concerned about how we would get both babies into the minivan, especially in the winter, and then drive them over to my mom's before work. My daughters didn't have the luxury of being carried in our arms whenever we arrived at our destination. My heart ached each time I'd see that they'd fallen asleep on our way somewhere. I hated that I'd have to wake them up so that they could walk in. Not only that, but sometimes they even carried their own diaper bags.

God always seemed to look out for us, though. Just as we were about to begin house shopping, we noticed that my mom's next-door neighbor had stopped sitting outside. One day while my mom was gardening and I was sitting with the girls, we saw a man mowing the neighbor's lawn. My mom asked me to interpret so she could find out where the kind little old lady had gone. I rolled over and got the man's attention. He turned off the lawnmower and I said, "My mom is concerned about the woman that lived in this house because she hasn't seen her all spring. Do you know if she is all right?" He said, "Oh, my aunt is no longer going to live here. She fell and we had to put her in a nursing home." I told my mom what the man had said, and my mom was saddened by the news. She said that she often went over to her house and helped her trim her bushes.

A lightbulb went on in my head, though. I quickly asked the neighbor's nephew, "What is happening to the house?" He said, "We are getting it ready to sell it." I said, "Can you hold on? I will be right back." I went inside and called Isidro, telling him that the house next door would soon be for sale. Isidro realized this could be exactly what we needed. He came outside and told the neighbor that we might be interested in the house. He asked, "Can we go in to see it?" The man wiped off his forehead and said, "It's a mess, but sure, you can come in to see it." We left the girls with my mom and entered the house.

It was shaped exactly like my mom's, a two-bedroom brick ranch home. Also like my parents' home, there was an addition on the back that included another bedroom, a bathroom, and a walk-in closet. There wasn't much sunlight coming in, though, because all the windows were covered with faded newspaper. The floors were covered with shaggy orange carpeting from the '70s. All the kitchen cabinets were probably original. We knew my mom's house was built in the 1950s, so the cabinets were likely to be over fifty years old. Many of the walls were made of paneling, and we noticed candles all over the place. The neighbor must have been religious because we saw a bunch of rosaries hanging throughout the house. My husband asked for the price and the man said they still had not decided. Isidro told him to please let us know as soon as they had a number in mind.

We went back to our home and discussed what we had seen. We realized that it would require a lot of updates and repairs, starting with remodeling the bathrooms and kitchen, removing the ugly orange carpeting, and replacing the dark paneling with brighter walls. Plus, we'd have to make several modifications to make it accessible for me. In any other situation, we would have not seen the potential, but the location was enough to convince us that the house would be ideal. What better home could we have found than one right next door to the girls' grandma and caregiver? We hoped that the price would be reasonable.

Within three months of first seeing it, we moved into our new home. The move was not difficult since we didn't have much furniture at my parents' house anyway. After financing and giving a down payment, we had some money left for purchasing furniture and making all the modifications. We hired several construction workers to do the work before we purchased the furniture. We only had a bed, the crib, the bassinet, basic essential dishes, and our clothes at the house until all the remodeling was done. In the end, we spent over $60,000 on all the changes.

Many of the changes required Franklin Park village permits. Obtaining some of them was difficult. We had to fight for them to allow us to build the ramp that was needed for me to be able to enter the house. At my parents', the back door was leveled, so I didn't have a problem getting in, especially because I could use the garage. But our new home had two small steps going up to it, which, for a wheelchair user, might as well have been a whole staircase. The village argued that they didn't want our home to look different from the rest of the houses. They hadn't counted on the fact I knew everything I did about the ADA, though. So, after some hassle, I was finally allowed to have a ramp built.

The location couldn't have been more ideal. In the morning, I would get ready for work and then call my mom to come to get the girls to take them to her house. She would take them in her arms, sometimes still asleep, to her house. Then, I would just leave to go to work. My mom would take care of them the whole day, sometimes for longer days, like when I had to stay late for a Harper event. The girls saw their grandma's house as an extension of their own home.

They had toys, clothes, and books in both residences. I paid mom to care for them and she would buy them what they liked to eat. They would have homemade meals that only my mom knew how to make. My mom was also watching Rique's daughter, Jennifer. The three girls were inseparable, even with their distinct personalities. While I was at work, sometimes I forgot to even check in on them. I was so fortunate to know that they were in loving hands.

I continued working with a wonderful team of caring professionals at Harper. I was building a strong, student-centered reputation at the college because I looked at the lives of students with disabilities holistically. I had the freedom to lead my colleagues in working on other projects and programs outside of ADS. For example, I was able to lead the department in organizing a "walk-n-roll" fundraising event to leverage support for starting a scholarship for students with disabilities. I solicited generous donations for t-shirts, pizza, and drinks for the participants. I collaborated with other areas of the college and held a very successful event that allowed us to meet our intended goal.

The college's foundation was very supportive of our initiatives. They allowed me to work on obtaining other donations that would continue to generate funding for the department. A friend, Lourdes, whom I'd met through Life Directions, worked for a home-decorating company. She informed me that the company was moving to another state and that they were donating all their goods. I wrote a request letter, and the company donated all their products to Harper. Of course, I had no idea of what I had gotten us into. It was no wonder that they verified that we would take all twenty pallets. I hadn't really realized the amount of merchandise they would be donating. Because Harper didn't know where to store the merchandise, I solicited the donation of a storage unit. In addition, I worked with custodial friends to help with the transport. We filled a 16 x 16 storage unit from floor to ceiling. I was overwhelmed with the amount of home decoration goods: ceramic decorations, dishes, frames, garden decorations, linens, and many other items. We had many internal sales of the items, and when the weather warmed up, we had our first (and only) garage sale in front of the Performing Arts Center. We had so much stuff that we decided to mark every item at the cheap price of one dollar. Beyond that, several of us agreed to have additional garage sales at our own homes. As a result, we earned over $30,000, which we used to start the ADS Alumni Scholarship, a Special Events Fund, and an Emergency Fund for students. Whatever items we had left after that year of various sales, we donated to Goodwill.

Raising two toddlers was fun, but difficult! My mom's support is what enabled Isidro and me to survive. They were smart babies and used each other for motivation. I recall the summer when Ariel was still two, but about to turn three in October, when we wanted to potty train her. Ariana had just turned two and she joined in the fun. She wanted to follow in her big sister's footsteps. Although my intent was only to potty train Ariel, I got two for the price of one. Within weeks, they got the hang of it, allowing us to get rid of diapers altogether. Our life became that much easier now that both were out of diapers.

They were active little girls, and we had vowed that they would live a full normal life despite our disabilities. This meant that we wanted our girls to experience and learn from every different kind of social activity. Even though at first we mostly played in the yard and went to parks, malls, and restaurants, as the years went on, they were frequent visitors to children's museums, Chuck E. Cheese and Enchanted Castle, Kiddieland (when it still existed), water parks, zoos, swimming pools, and outdoor parks. Ariel and Ariana learned to be very independent from an early age. They relied on each other for companionship and our encouragement to risk doing new activities.

I will admit that, to entertain them, I probably contributed my fair share of pollution. They loved balloons. One time I got them a balloon, and when Ariel let it go, I thought she would start to cry. She didn't, and instead waved at the flying balloon, saying, "Bye, bye balloon." Ariana always copied her older sister, so she also began waving goodbye to the balloon. I got such a kick out of it that I decided to buy a helium tank and blow balloons so they could let them go.

Of course, I didn't count on this becoming a family tradition. They clamored and demanded more "bye, bye balloons."

When we did venture out into the public, we would be a sight to see. People couldn't fathom how two parents with disabilities had not one but two girls. We would load them into their double stroller, pushed by me. I became a pro in maneuvering my wheelchair with one hand while pushing the double stroller with the other. We wanted to be out and about and didn't want them secluded at home, although we would only venture to places where we thought we could control their safety. I didn't want them to feel targeted by any stares, so I would say, "They are looking because they really like your stroller" or "They are looking because they like my wheelchair." Their self-esteem was not impacted negatively by the reactions of strangers.

One time, we underestimated their angelic faces. When in public places, Isidro and I didn't let them walk around for fear of them running off. Usually we would tie them to their seats on their double stroller and not let them out. We went to a nearby mall when they were about two or three years old. They were behaving well, looking calmly at the people walking around. Isidro told me, "They have been good. They are probably tired of sitting, so let's let them walk for a bit." I responded, "Are you sure we should do that?" He was already unbuckling Ariel as he responded, "Yes." First, he got Ariel out, who stood still watching as Ariana was being taken out. As soon as Ariana was out, though, it was as if permission had been granted for Ariel to take off running. If I didn't know better, I would have thought they planned the whole thing, because, soon after, Ariana took off running too. Of course, to make it even more challenging, each of them ran off in different directions. Isidro started walking fast after Ariel, while I zoomed to try to catch Ariana.

The chase included an obstacle course. Ariana entered a Victoria's Secret store and because the display tables were so high and she was so tiny, she didn't even have to duck to slip underneath them and evade my capture. The other shoppers didn't know whether to laugh or help us. Of course, Isidro was having his own challenges. All I heard was him yelling, "Ariel, come back!" Finally, strangers came to the rescue and helped us trap them. By this time, we were sweating. We didn't even have time to be embarrassed since we were totally occupied with trying to regain our control. We were so exhausted after all the excitement that we quit shopping and went straight home.

My girls were usually compliant, but, as normal toddlers, they did have their bouts with the Terrible Twos. I discovered a great way to allow them to walk while still controlling how far off they went. It was a vest with buckles that had a long belt for me to hold on to; it was like having them on a leash. Although at first I was bothered by the concept of holding on to them like I would hold on to a dog, I learned to love having the harness. Isidro and I would each hold one of the girls as we shopped. On one certain shopping excursion, everything had run smoothly until we were leaving the store and heading to our car. I am not sure what it was that Ariana wanted to do, but she didn't want to leave. I tried to direct her by lightly tugging the cord for her to follow. She was not happy and decided to have her first ever temper tantrum right in the middle of the road. She began crying and threw herself on the ground, wailing loudly. I tried to lift her, but I was afraid that my wheelchair would topple over. Isidro quickly loaded Ariel into the minivan and came to help me as I tried to protect her from cars. She proved that indeed she was a normal two-year-old.

They were so blessed to have the nurturing love of Mama China and Papa Lalo (as they learned to call my parents). My mom spoiled them by cooking their favorite foods, including foods that she probably shouldn't have given them. As young as three, they were given coffee as part of their breakfast. When I found out, I thought I should talk to my mom about it. I said, "Mom, I don't think it's a good idea to give them coffee because of the caffeine." She replied, "Oh, don't worry, it is more milk than coffee. Nothing will happen to them." The girls learned that the rules in my home were different than in grandma's home. I didn't let them drink soda, but my mom would sometimes give them RC or Sprite in their bottles.

Speaking of bottles, I was proud because I thought I had done a good job weaning them off bottles when they were toddlers. Of course, they were weaned in my house but not in their other home. I think they continued drinking "tetes" until they were almost school aged. Hey, the pink Nesquik was pretty good! I think I could have gotten hooked on it too. Ariana not only loved her bottles, but she couldn't live without her pacifiers. Ariel preferred sucking her blankie, the one I met her in. I was getting concerned about the addiction to their vices, but when I asked the pediatrician, he downplayed it and said, "Trust me, when they start school they won't want to drink from a bottle or suck on a blankie."

Admittedly, both addictions were probably my fault. In my head, I wanted Ariel to have a piece of her birth mom because I wanted her to grow up feeling nurtured. I would always give her the blanket and she started soothing herself with it. First, she would cover her face with it and then eventually graduated to sucking it. I was equally guilty about Ariana's love for pacifiers. I knew she loved them, so I began to buy the pacifiers to match her outfits. She ended up with quite the collection both in our home and in my mom's. After years of sucking on a binky, she couldn't be without one. I began to feel embarrassed that she would always have one stuck in her mouth. At least Ariel just used her blanket at night, but Ariana was always hooked on the pacifier.

When Ariana was about four, I wanted to register her for the same preschool that Ariel was attending, but I wanted her weaned off the binkies. In our roles as parents, I was always the bad cop while Isidro was the lenient one. Anytime I would try to take away the pacifier, Isidro would cave in and give it back to her. Isidro had not seen his parents and sisters for a few years, so we decided that he should take a trip to Austin alone, since the girls were still too young. I used this time as my opportunity to get rid of the pacifiers once and for all. I decided to use her intelligence for my plan. I announced to both girls, "We are going to do an art project." They got excited and waited for directions. I said, "Find all the pacifiers and bring them here to the coffee table." Eagerly, they looked for all the pacifiers. I helped them by pointing out where there might be other pacifiers. Once they had all the pacifiers, about twenty of them, I gave them each a pair of children's scissors. I said, "OK, we are going to cut all the pacifiers like this." I modeled how to cut the rubber off into small pieces. Ariana and Ariel wanted to compete, so they quickly began cutting. It didn't take long for all the pacifiers to be in pieces.

The next part of the craft was to glue the pieces of rubber onto a piece of art paper. I suggested they make a sun or a moon out of them. They were thrilled, trying to come up with the best picture. Each of them created their own individual masterpiece. They glowed with pride, especially when I took them to hang on the refrigerator. They had smiles from ear to ear. We then cleaned up the mess and had dinner. They kept looking at their designs, saying, "Bonito!" I would agree and compliment them each on the great job they did.

At bedtime, they took their baths and I had them choose which book they each wanted as a nighttime story. We had set up their room with twin beds so that I could go between each bed to give them individual attention. As I read Ariel's story, I could see Ariana getting restless. I said, "What's wrong, Ariana?" She said, "Chupon," the Spanish word for pacifier. I said, "No hay." I reminded her that there were no more pacifiers. She started to get upset but I reminded her of the beautiful pictures they had made with their chupones. I got them up and took them to the kitchen to savor their beautiful pieces of art once again. As we looked at the pictures, I said, "See, your pacifiers are now beautiful pieces of art." She had no option but to accept that her binkies were all gone and that she had participated in their destruction. I put them in bed and turned off the light. I didn't hear crying, so I felt good that my plan had worked.

In the morning, as soon as she got up, Ariana went to the kitchen to look at her art. This time it wasn't with a smile but rather with disappointment. She accepted that they were gone and there was nothing that could be done about it. After breakfast we went out to the yard for them to play. They ran around in the yard greeting my dad who was mowing the yards. My dad went to trim one of the bushes and saw a squirrel who had gotten stuck and died. He pulled it out as I guarded the girls from getting too close and looked at the dead animal. I explained that the squirrel went to heaven.

The girls were content with my explanation and continued playing. A few minutes later, Ariana ran to me excitedly and announced, "Mami, I found a chupon." She had probably dropped it a previous day. I immediately had to react because I didn't want to go back to step one now that she had had at least one night without a pacifier. I said, "Quick, give it to me. I have to throw it out because the squirrel tried to eat it and that is why it died." With a shocked face, Ariana quickly handed it to me and watched as I threw it in the trash. That was the end of the pacifier addiction.

My dad, their Papa Lalo, also spoiled them. He would go to a small grocery store near our home and buy them ice cream. My dad was nearly eighty, but in good health apart from neuropathy caused by his previous stroke. He came home and gave each girl an ice cream bar. The three of them sat on the front step, him in the middle with one girl on each side, eating their treats. They loved Papa Lalo, though Ariana, who was starting to show her shy personality, wouldn't often show that love. My dad would beg for her to give him a kiss, and she would just turn around. On the other hand, Ariel was very affectionate and kissed him and everyone on demand.

Life was hectic, so I didn't always make the time I should have to have conversations with my dad. We talked, but usually they were routine conversations. I learned that his greatest attribute was gratefulness. One day, while he was outside mowing his lawn, I took the girls outside to play. In the front of my house, we have a big magnolia tree. Ariana, my little monkey, loved climbing it. She climbed with ease and went to the topmost branch. I had stopped worrying because she was a true acrobat. My dad suddenly stopped the lawnmower in the middle of his lawn. He came to me and said, "God is great." I responded, "Yes he is." He said, "Look at Ariana up there. Can you believe she was born from you?" I turned to look at her and just waited for him to continue. He said, "What we would've given for you to be able to climb a tree. But now God has given that ability to your daughter." I said, "Yes, she is doing what I was never able to do." Convincingly he said, "We should always thank God for the blessings he gives us even if we have to wait." He then went back to his lawnmower. I sat there with an even deeper appreciation for the miracle God had given me, up there in that magnolia tree.

Another decision we made as parents was to try to raise Ariel and Ariana as fully bilingual. When they were little, Isidro and I would only talk to them in Spanish unless we slipped and spoke in English. They of course also knew Spanish thanks to spending so much time with my parents. My mom never learned English, and my dad knew some but preferred Spanish. But we knew that once they started school, it would be more challenging to maintain the Spanish. I even attempted to have them enrolled in the bilingual program, but because Isidro and I both knew English, they didn't accept them into the program. I hoped that both girls would maintain their culture even after entering school.

When the girls finally started school, my dad would walk them to the corner and wait for the bus to pick them up. Later in the afternoon, regardless of the weather, he would be out there again, waiting for them to get home, standing there as if he had not moved the whole day. The girls never fussed about not wanting to go to school, so I never worried about them missing the bus or not finding someone waiting for them when they got home. I counted on my dad as much as I counted on my mom.

My parents and I didn't always agree with what we believed was best for my girls. But for the most part, I trusted fully that my parents knew what they were doing, so I didn't make a big deal over my mom giving the girls coffee or soda. However, when it came to what I thought was best for Ariel in terms of her adoption, I didn't compromise. From the very beginning, I wanted both girls to know the truth about their births. I always talked to Ariel about the day I met her in Mexico. I didn't want to risk her finding out about her adoption from someone else.

My mom and dad were concerned and thought that I shouldn't tell her because it might affect her negatively. I explained to my parents that psychologists recommended that we be open about the adoption. I explained that I had researched this topic and concluded that Ariel would be better off knowing the truth. I knew that as a child she was not going to understand what it meant, but I hoped she would become familiar with the story and feel safe to ask questions when she grew older. Similarly, I wanted Ariana to know the truth and to understand how they were both equally loved by the entire family.

Besides reading books about adoption and other types of topics of diversity, I wanted to read books about parents with disabilities. I searched and the only books on disability that I found were very patronizing. Children's books on disability usually referred to disabled people as "special." They depicted people with disabilities as needy and dependent. I wasn't pleased with these portrayals or with the minimal selection of books covering this topic. I thought to myself, I want books where disability is normalized. I didn't want my girls to feel less than because both parents had disabilities.

As I often do, I don't just complain, but I try to solve my problems. Because of my love for writing, I decided to write a children's book. After finishing *My Mom Rocks; Her Chair Rolls*, a former sociology professor from DePaul who had started a publishing company agreed to put it out. On the verge of printing the book, unfortunately, he encountered financial difficulties and his company had to close. Regardless, I still read the book to the girls because it portrayed the type of image I wanted them to have regarding parents with disabilities. Here is the beginning of the book:

Our Mom Rocks; Her Chair Rolls

Our mom rocks; her chair rolls.
We love her so much with all our souls.
Not on two feet, but on her seat
She is someone you want to meet!

Both girls were always in the same grade, although we always requested that they attend different classrooms. We wanted to avoid any competition since we observed their different strengths and struggles. Ariel was a social butterfly and loved making friends. She didn't struggle walking up to a child to ask, "Want to be my friend?" She also had a heart of gold. One time at the circus, I had bought her an elephant-shaped cup and because we were seated in the handicapped section, there was a child in a wheelchair nearby. Ariel walked over to the kid and said, "Want my cup?" She was so kind that I would often call her "My Mother Theresa." She was always willing to try new things even if she was not graceful in them. Ariel seemed to struggle more with reading, but she was an expert socially. I knew her social skills would help her out in life.

Ariana, on the other hand, had been an introvert since she was very young. She preferred to be alone or to just play with her sister. She was very shy and never talked, even among other kids. She spoke at home where she was comfortable, but as soon as we were in a public place, it was as if someone had taped her mouth shut. She was so bright, though, that sometimes it would get her into trouble. I still remember how, using nail polish, she put her name on every DVD that she owned. Of course, she did this under Isidro's watch.

Ariana was also stubborn! No matter what activity I signed her up for, she didn't want to participate. It was maddening that, during her gymnastics class, she would refuse to participate, yet she happily did the gymnastics stunts on our way home. She was always running her own race. She didn't succumb to peer pressure. If she liked something, there was no changing her mind. Once when we went to buy her new shoes, she liked a certain pair and no matter what other ones I suggested, she had already made up her mind. The issue, though, was that the pair she wanted were for the same foot. The clerk and I looked all over for the other shoe but were unsuccessful. She didn't care. To teach her a lesson, I bought the pair. Soon she realized that they were not too comfortable. Of course, I'd kept the receipt.

Ariana was too smart for her own good. One night, after the night routine, I laid them in their beds, turned off the light, turned on the night light, and shut the door. By nine, it was all lights out, and I would wind down in my bedroom until I went to sleep. Almost at ten, my mom called. I panicked when I saw her name on the caller ID. I quickly answered and said, "Is everything all right?" She said, "Did you lose something valuable today?" Confused, I said, "Like what?" She answered and said, "Like something little, worth a million bucks." I still had no idea what she was talking about. I said, "Not that I know of." She said, "Well, Ariana is here having cookies and milk." I said, "What? I had her in bed!" She said, "Don't worry, I will let her finish and walk her back."

Good thing we lived in a good neighborhood. I couldn't believe she had walked next door all by herself and that I had no idea she had done so. When she got home, I scolded her and told her she couldn't do that again. However, her nocturnal outings didn't stop even after we put a chain on the door. She just moved over her little bathroom step stool and, with the stick of the broom, managed to take off the chain. She loved going to my mom's. I kept explaining the dangers, but that didn't deter her. I finally told her, just let me know when you're going so I can call my mom and watch you go. Her visits were usually short, and I didn't want to fight this battle.

Ariana wasn't much older when she announced that she was running away. I hadn't let her start watching a movie because I wanted to go outside with them. She wasn't happy. She grabbed her rolling princess suitcase and started packing it, announcing, "I'm running away." I said, "Make sure you don't forget anything." With a pout, she said, "I didn't." I asked, "Do you have your toothbrush?" She didn't answer but ran to the bathroom. She placed her toothbrush in the suitcase and zipped it up. She opened the door and started walking out. I said, "I will miss you!" She continued on her path, but then Ariel lost it! She started crying, telling me not to let her sister go. I calmed her down by telling her, "Let's go tell Mama China to get Ariana."

My mom was outside and wondered where Ariana was going with the suitcase but just assumed that she was playing. I almost wanted to laugh when I saw Ariana at the end of the block, standing there without moving. She was still not allowed to cross the street alone. When I explained to my mom what was going on, she said, "Let me go get her." I don't know what she told her, but Ariana came back with her and forgot why she was mad in the first place.

The girls learned to help with chores much younger than most other kids did. Ariana learned to do laundry before she even started school. Because my washer wasn't accessible, and I couldn't reach the clothes after they were washed, Ariana would get inside the washer and take all the clothes out. She learned quickly how to sort by color. She began to do laundry on her own in elementary school. Plus, they helped by getting up on the counters to get items down from the cabinets. Ariana was very agile and managed to reach anything I needed.

Sometimes others questioned why I allowed them to do things that other kids their age never did. Once, we were shopping and I wanted to see a pair of flip-flops for the girls, but they were up too high. So, I told Ariana to climb on my lap, then up onto my chair so she could reach them. One of the clerks saw this and came over. She said, "Ma'am, you shouldn't endanger your child like that." Being a bit perturbed, without thinking I said, "She is my child and I can endanger her if I want." I quickly realized what I'd just said and corrected myself, saying that she was perfectly safe or else I wouldn't have allowed her to climb on me. The clerk left all flustered.

Growing up with parents with disabilities, our girls had a different type of childhood, but I know that different doesn't necessarily mean worse. I hoped the skills they learned as children would help them later in life. Although it was difficult to believe that we had successfully raised them to be school-aged children, I kept reminding myself: bigger kids, bigger problems. But I was still content to enter this new stage of life.

I don't know if I was too busy to notice or what, but I was struggling physically. I started to experience body aches and pains. I also noticed that I was losing strength in my arms. What I used to be able to do, now I couldn't. I was also extremely fatigued and couldn't understand why. At work, I was struggling more and more physically, although not mentally. Mentally, I was stronger than ever. I had so many ideas and just not enough time to implement them all. As Coordinator of Learning Services, I didn't want my disability to interfere with my life again. However, I knew better. I knew that I would find a solution for whatever was next in my life. I just prayed that along with the tears there would be sunshine.

CHAPTER 21

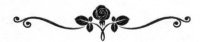

I
t was incredible how fast the girls were growing. From the beginning, they were opposites, but I was glad that they loved each other and that they got along like best friends. Ariel was having academic difficulties, and I saw how challenging school was for her. Ariana was doing well in all her classes, but the teachers complained that she wouldn't talk. I told the teachers that she talked at home, but still, they always raised a concern.

Perhaps because of my experience in the field of disability services, I suspected that Ariel might have a disability because of her struggles with reading, spelling, and writing. The school, though, preferred to give her interventions instead of testing her. When she had the interventions, she seemed to improve, but as soon as they were removed, she struggled again. I noticed problems with anything that dealt with language. Sometimes I saw her struggle even with speaking. She said, "Mom, I can't find my thingy." I asked, "What thing?" She tried to recall the name of the thing as if it were on the tip of her tongue but wouldn't come out. She responded, "You know, the thing." It was frustrating for her and equally difficult for me.

Ariel was always compliant and didn't miss school, though it was obvious that it was difficult for her. Plus, she seemed anxious all the time. She would freak out if she lost sight of me at the store. She could never go to a different aisle because she would become overly anxious. She was also anxious at night. From a very young age, she would ensure that all the doors were locked, even double locked. God forbid that a shade was left opened. She wanted all the windows locked, secure, and with the blinds down. Since I never met her birth mother or knew anything about her, I didn't know if this anxiety ran in her family. Her grades were always Cs and Ds. But the comments always spoke about her friendliness and willingness to help.

On the other hand, Ariana did well academically but struggled socially. She seemed to get in trouble because of her intelligence and unwillingness to speak up. While at work, when Ariana was in first grade, I received a call from her teacher. She wanted to report that Ariana had gone under all the bathroom stalls and locked them. According to her teacher, she found Ariana laughing because the girls had to go to the bathroom but couldn't because the stalls were locked.

I couldn't believe that Ariana had done that because she was shy but not mean. In the evening, when I questioned Ariana, she said that she didn't lock the bathroom stalls. She insisted that they were already closed when they went in and that she went under to unlock them. However, she did admit to laughing when a girl kept trying to get into a stall but couldn't. I asked, "Why didn't you tell your teacher?" She just shrugged her shoulders. I said, "Would you like if someone laughed if you couldn't get into a bathroom stall and had an accident?" She said, "No." I said, "Well, I want you to say sorry to the little girl. I will also call your teacher about what really happened. In the meantime, you are on time out so you can have time to think about what happened today."

She had another altercation with her second-grade teacher. She was getting all As, but her teacher kept commenting on Ariana not talking and not answering when she was asked a direct question. Again, her teacher called to complain about Ariana's behavior. She said, "Ariana took some Rice Krispie Treats from the snack cabinet." The teacher explained that the students had been explicitly told not to grab any snacks without permission. Again, I was surprised that I was getting another complaint about her.

I also was surprised because we had Rice Krispie Treats at home. I always bought them for quick snacks, but she rarely ate them. I knew we had some at home, so I couldn't understand why she would grab one without permission. I told the teacher I would discuss this with Ariana and handle it appropriately. I called my mom during my lunch and told her that Ariana's teacher had called and complained about Ariana taking a Rice Krispie Treat. My mom wasn't happy, but not at Ariana but at the teacher for making a big deal about a snack. She said, "What does she think? It's like leaving a bottle of tequila for an alcoholic and expecting him not to drink it." I said, "Well, it's wrong to take something that doesn't belong to her." She said, "Kids are innocent. She is just a bitter lady."

When I got home, I asked Ariana, "What happened today at school?" She said, "Nothing." I said, "Well, your teacher called me and said you took a Rice Krispie Treat without permission. Did you?" She said, "All my friends did." I asked, "Why did you do it?" She said, "Because my friends told me to do it." I asked, "Did you tell the teacher that?" She shrugged her shoulders. I asked again, "Did you tell your teacher that your friends told you to grab one?" She said no. I said, "You deserve a punishment because you listened to your friends and took something you shouldn't have." Her eyes opened wide and said, "Am I on time out?" I said, "No, tomorrow you are going to take a box of Rice Krispie Treats to your teacher and tell her you are sorry." She didn't think this was a bad punishment until I said she had to pay me back for the Rice Krispie Treats with extra chores.

My life was consumed with my two fast growing kids and my job. I was constantly on the go. I started feeling more exhausted than ever. I couldn't figure out why. Winters were especially difficult for me. There were days that it was a complete sacrifice to get up and go to work. However, I always pushed through my aches. One winter, during our break, we got a lot of snow, and I got so discouraged because my aches became worse because of it. Though my dad had begun to slow down, he still insisted on clearing the snow from our path. One day after he did so, he came in and sat on my living room sofa. I was in the kitchen but could see him while I was cooking breakfast. He said, "I just cleared your snow. It was heavy today." I said, "Dad, I can't believe that you chose to bring us here to Chicago when you could have chosen Florida or California." With a somber expression he said, "You have done well in Chicago." I replied, "Yes, but I would have been happier with better weather." He slowly got up while I continued with my dish. He said, "I am leaving." I said, "OK, thank you for clearing the snow."

Later in the day, my mom came over and said, "What happened?" With confusion I asked, "About what?" She said, "Your dad is very hurt about what you said." I asked, "What did I say?" She tells me that my dad was offended because I told him he should not have brought us to Chicago. Laughing I said, "You got to be kidding me. Look at the weather outside. I hate living here." She said, "But your dad sacrificed a lot to get us to Chicago. You should say sorry." Stubbornly I said, "I don't think I was rude or disrespectful. I was giving him my opinion, and he should have understood." My mom said, "You know your dad feels proud, especially because you are so successful." I said, "I know, and I will always be grateful, but I still don't think I did anything wrong by telling him how I feel about snow." She let it go, got up, and left, and we never talked about it again.

My attitude reflected how I was feeling physically, though. I wondered if all the aches and pain were indications that the polio was coming back? I tried to look for information about polio, but it was scarce. However, I found information about a condition called Post-Polio Syndrome, and it was clear that I was experiencing all the symptoms described. I talked to my primary doctor and pursued going to a specialist. I received a referral to see a specialist, Dr. Seever, who worked at Rush Hospital in Chicago. It felt good to see a doctor who had been a leader during the polio epidemic in the 1950s in Chicago. It was so interesting to learn from him all about the devastating damage that polio had caused. He confirmed that I was experiencing Post-Polio. He said, "Your fatigue, your body aches, your pain, and your muscle weakness are due to Post-Polio Syndrome." I asked him if there were any treatments, and his response was one word: "Rest."

Dr. Seever was probably in his 80s, but I felt entirely confident in what he was telling me. I felt understood. I'd started to worry and kept telling myself, *Come on; you've never been lazy.* But talking to him allowed me to understand that I wasn't going crazy; rather, my symptoms were because of the damage polio caused over the forty years before. Besides his knowledge, I enjoyed his humor. He told me that all the polio survivors he knew were type-A personalities. I chuckled and said, "But not me." He responded, "Yeah, sure." He explained the science behind the symptoms I was experiencing, which explained why after any physical activity such as grocery shopping, doing laundry, or cooking, I felt unable to move. It felt so good to speak to someone who truly comprehended what I was living through.

He told me, "You need to slow down. You have already won all the medals. You don't have to prove yourself to anyone." I said, "But I work and have two daughters." He said, "Do you want to live independently?" I responded, "Of course!" With a serious expression he said, "At your rate, you will lose your independence in ten years. You must slow down." He asked if I was getting any accommodations at work. I told him that I didn't need any. He said, "Of course you do. You need a reduced schedule so you can rest." I told him that he'd given me a lot to think about and that I would look for solutions. Thanks to seeing this doctor, I did finally make some changes.

It's funny how I had worked in helping students find accommodations, but I had never asked for any accommodations for myself. Now with the ADA, though, things were different, and access was a legal right I had. Throughout my schooling, I had learned how to accommodate myself by finding solutions and advocating for myself. It's no wonder that I'd done the same at Harper. I decided that I wanted to be around for my girls, though, so I had to make changes.

I asked for the accommodation of being able to work one day from home. Tom, who was always very understanding, didn't have an issue with my request. He knew it was reasonable and that I was a hard worker and wasn't taking advantage. However, he suggested I make it official by making the request through human resources. In 2006, I was diagnosed with Post-Polio Syndrome and given the accommodation to work from home on Wednesdays.

Aside from getting approval to work from home one day a week, I also changed the type of wheelchair I used. Dr. Seever had stressed that I should not push my body or else it might give up and no longer want to work. I always ignored pain and just accomplished what I had to do without paying attention to my fatigue, body aches, or pain. But I had to change how I got around at Harper. I decided to start using a motorized wheelchair, which meant I would also have to change the type of vehicle I drove. It was a big decision and I put it off for as long as I could. For some reason, I'd thought that if I started using a powered wheelchair, it meant that I had given up. I had no idea, though, that the power wheelchair would give me so much more freedom than I ever could have imagined.

The cost of a modified van is almost twice as expensive as a regular minivan. But it had to be modified so that I could ride up the ramp and transfer into the driver's seat, in addition to installing the standard hand controls I used. The first minivan I purchased cost $63,000. I was shocked by the price and even more shocked to find out that there was no financial support available to offset the cost. The only offer was from General Motors, who gave individuals with disabilities a $1,000 rebate. We had to refinance our home to take out some of the equity from the property for the purchase. Fortunately, my insurance covered the cost of my motorized wheelchair. It was worth it, though—it was fabulous driving to places and not needing to be pushed. I zoomed around quickly without the strenuous damage to my arm muscles. After I experienced the benefits, my concerns over powered chairs dissipated.

Working Wednesdays from home was great, though I stressed myself wanting to prove that I was working. I always said that I worked harder at home than I did when I was on campus. At home, there were no distractions like catching up with colleagues about their personal lives or being interrupted by people who just had a quick question. I cranked up my laptop bright and early and worked nonstop on all the projects that I was involved in. During this time, I also thought about ideas for other programs that would help support students.

Because the US economy was not doing well, we'd experienced a decline in students signing up for the fee-for-service tutoring program. So I wrote a proposal to take a sabbatical leave that would allow me to do research on how to better serve students by finding out what motivated them. My application was approved, so I went on a semester-long leave. I visited all the high schools within Harper's district and did presentations to groups of students with disabilities. I spoke to audiences ranging in size from ten to five hundred; my public speaking skills improved tremendously during this time.

I also gave presentations at the churches in my area. I shared my story and the importance of faith. One day while grocery shopping, a woman approached me and said, "You changed my life." I had no clue what she was talking about, so I asked, "Do you know me?" She said, "I listened to your story at my church." She continued, "You shared your experiences with your pregnancies and how you adopted a child." I said, "Yes, I was blessed." She said, "Thank you. When I was listening to you, I had just found out that I was pregnant." I stopped in the middle of the grocery isle and listened intently. She then said, "I was pregnant and thinking of having an abortion, but after all that you went through, I realized that it would be a mistake to abort." She then pointed to the baby in her cart and said, "She is here because of you." I was speechless and thanked God for using me as an instrument to help this woman.

My dad had taken a fall on the 4th of July and broke his hip. Similar to my own experience, he'd broken it without doing anything dangerous. He was sitting in the kitchen, taking his medications when he dropped a pill. When he bent down to get it, he slipped off his chair and broke his hip. He had a successful hip replacement, but for some reason he developed dementia while in the hospital. We didn't know if it was because of the anesthesia or because of the painkillers he was on. He came home after he was discharged from the hospital, but he was totally incapacitated.

My nephew Adrian, Mon's son, had studied to be a certified nursing assistant, so he agreed to help with my dad's recuperation. He needed constant care because he risked falling every time he attempted to get up. Because my sabbatical offered flexibility in my schedule, I also had time to go visit my dad. God is clearly always looking out for me. I was so saddened when my dad started losing his memory and didn't recognize me. I left his house crying one day because he asked, "Who are you?" I said, "It's me Cuali, your daughter." He responded, "No you aren't. Cuali had short hair, and you have long hair." When I lived with him, I'd had short hair for the most part. I had just let it grow within the past few years. I was so upset that I went home and picked up a pair of scissors, just like the time I fell when I was in college and cut my hair after. I wanted my dad to recognize me. I loved him so much.

My concern was not only for my dad's health, but also for my mom's well-being. She was not getting enough sleep and was worrying about my dad constantly. I knew that she was fearing the end of my dad's life, and I feared the same because he was not improving. His hip appeared to have healed, but he was still unable to walk and his mind was more confused than ever. My God decided to call him home on December 15, 2007—thirty-six years to the day that he had first brought us all to Chicago. He died with everyone around his bed, surrounded by his greatest treasure, his family. For years, the memory of that conversation we once had during the winter came to mind. I felt horrible and so guilty for never having apologized for asking him why he'd brought us to Chicago. I wanted him to know how grateful I was, but it was too late. My dad was a magnificent man. The many lessons he taught us would live on throughout our lives.

We held his wake, funeral, and burial shortly after his death. We were devastated to lose a man who had given his whole life to support his family in obtaining the American dream. For years I had kept the small heart-shaped ceramic container with my son Cristian's ashes. I had never figured out an appropriate place to disperse the remains, so I just kept them in our living room curio cabinet. Without discussing it with anyone, not even Isidro, I took the precious container to my dad's wake. When I rolled up and saw him in the casket, so many thoughts flooded my mind. He looked so dignified in the three-piece suit he had worn to his anniversary celebration. I grabbed the little ceramic heart and laid it by his hands. I silently said a small prayer and said, "Dad, watch over your grandson. Cristian, watch over your grandpa." I knew my son couldn't be in better hands. This brought me peace for many years to come. Now they would have each other.

My girls were too little to understand what had happened. However, they recognized that my mom was extremely sad. I was worried about my mom being alone, so I talked to Isidro and asked if he would be OK with the girls sleeping at my mom's house for a while so she wouldn't be so lonely. He agreed with my idea, but I also wanted to make sure that the girls would want to do that as well. I talked to them and said, "Ariel and Ariana, Mama China is all alone in her house. Papa Lalo went to heaven. Do you want to sleep there to keep her company?" Ariel asked, "Is she afraid?" I responded, "No. She is just sad." They both said, "Yes. We don't want Mama China to be sad." I called my mom and asked her if she'd like for the girls to go over and sleep there. She welcomed them with open arms. Every evening after work, I'd pick them up and bring them to our place to do homework, eat dinner, take baths, and get ready for bed. Then once they were ready, they'd run next door. At first, I thought this would only last for a few weeks, but both the girls and my mom wanted it to be a permanent arrangement. I just hoped that I was not making a mistake.

Based on all the research and work I did during my sabbatical leave, I formulated an idea for a new program that would be a substitute for the PASS program we'd started at Harper in 1993. I recommended that new students enroll in a targeted class that prepared them for college, where the person who taught the course would also become an academic coach for the student. I showed how, instead of just bringing in program fees, the students would now be bringing in tuition money. The Academic Coaches Empowering Students (ACES) program began in the Fall of 2008 and still exists today. I remained one of the faculty members who taught the course, First Year Experience (FYE101), and added those students to my caseload.

We subsequently did extensive outcomes assessments for ACES and the results were very positive. Students with disabilities who were in ACES tended to be more successful. The retention rates and GPA were higher for students in the program than for those who were not. For a few years, I also taught a class for students with various disabilities alongside my friend Stacey, a counselor who taught a section for students on the autism spectrum. We developed the curriculum together and had a lot of fun. At first, we didn't know how it would turn out. But after a successful first year, we saw the benefits for both populations. The students on the autism spectrum were able to see appropriate social behavior from my students with other disabilities, and the students in my section, who had a variety of disabilities including learning disabilities, attention deficit disorder, anxiety, and depression, were able to see the high academic performance of the students who they might otherwise just see as "odd behaving." This proved to be just as rewarding an experience for Stacey and myself as it was for the students.

Stacey and I also traveled to conferences together to share our experience with teaching these targeted classes. She often said that she learned more from watching me deal with the lack of access than she did at the conference panels themselves. She was shocked at the ignorance of others when they interacted with me. For instance, a PhD professional sitting at our table at a conference once said, "How do students react to you when they see you in a wheelchair?" Stacey couldn't believe that woman had the guts to ask such a stupid question, especially when she didn't know me. Another professional at the conference said, "I saw someone else in a scooter; maybe the two of you can race." I had warned Stacey what it would be like traveling with me. But what surprised her more was that I didn't get offended, or at least, I didn't show I was offended.

During one of our conferences in Florida, Stacey was determined to get me to sit out at the beach with her. I told her that I normally couldn't go because wheelchairs tend to dig into the sand, making it impossible for me or anyone else to push. But without telling me, she did some research and found out about special wheelchairs for the sand. She said, "We are going to the beach! I rented you a hot rod." I was able to transfer into it, and she pushed me onto the sand. The wheelchair had large air tires that didn't sink in. I loved it, though it was extremely hot. We sat, and for the first time, I was one in the crowd. After a couple of hours, we went back to where I had left my own chair. I tried to transfer but couldn't. Probably because of heat exhaustion, I felt weak. She saw me struggling, so she said, "Let me get someone to help."

Stacey scouted out the best candidate. She saw a tall African American man dressed nicely in business casual attire. She said, "Sir, my friend is struggling to get into her wheelchair. Do you mind helping?" The gentleman replied, "I am a guest at the hotel. I don't work here." Stacey smiled and said, "Oh, I was just asking because you look strong." The man felt embarrassed because he'd thought Stacey had assumed he was probably a bellhop just because he was Black. After that awkward situation, he felt obligated to help. I used his arm for leverage and was able to transfer.

Debbie, another colleague from Harper, was also a frequent traveler to conferences with me. We have millions of examples of the challenges I faced because of my physical disability. For starters, it was challenging for me to board an airplane. I was usually assisted by airport staff and seated on the aisle, where only half of my behind could fit. It was kind of like being loaded into the plane like a piece of luggage. Then we had constant problems with hotel rooms, which were supposed to be accessible and yet the bed was somehow always super high or the shower would have no seat. Even with these challenges, though, we had a ball. Sometimes a bag of popcorn and a box of chocolate was all we needed. It certainly made up for not having access to the hotel's facilities such as the swimming pool. One of the best trips we took was to New Mexico, where we went to see the yearly air balloon show. (Don't be mistaken—we attended the conference; it wasn't all just fun and sightseeing!)

Even on Harper's campus, I experienced my share of microaggressions from otherwise well-meaning staff. I have many examples, but the ones that bothered me most include:

- Being told that I am lucky because I don't have to wear uncomfortable high heels. (If they only knew what happened when I tried a pair.)
- Coming to a meeting when someone says, "Oh, we have a wheelchair here. We weren't expecting one." (What about me? Were you expecting the PERSON in the chair?)
- Being asked if someone could hang their coat on my wheelchair. (As far as I know, I am not a coat rack.)
- Being invited to a faculty event that had been scheduled on the second floor of a building without an elevator. (Oops, I should have known better than to try to be social with my colleagues.)

These things really happened to me. Most of the time, I wasn't bothered. However, each incident chips away at a piece of me, leaving scars that often do not heal. Even though Stacey, Debbie, and many others might believe that situations that lack access don't bother me, they would be incorrect. Each time I go through a difficult situation, it's another injury to my confidence or self-esteem. Over time, I've learned how to push forward and not focus on my feelings. However, when I am alone and remember the hurtful incidents, I sometimes cry. But perhaps because my mom modeled for me how to be strong, I've been able to survive and continue. I never allow myself too much time to dwell on the hurt. I've always moved on because I had something else to accomplish!

Ariel and Ariana were used to my traveling and working hard. Still, they were realizing that our family was unique. They knew that access had to be figured out for us whenever we went to a public event, and they were used to us being spectators rather than participants at many of their events. But we still got them involved in everything. They participated in gymnastics, karate, baseball, violin playing, piano playing, and altar serving, to name a few. We also had them try out things that we'd never experienced. Whenever they were hesitant to try something out, I would say, "Please do it because I never have." For example, Ariana was unsure about riding a horse, but I convinced her when I said, "Please get on the horse and tell me about it because I've never been on one before."

We had our fifteen minutes of fame when ABC-TV did a news story on our family. A reporter who aired a weekly report on topics of disability interviewed us after I contacted her to see if she could do a positive story about parenting when disabled. She arranged for her camera crew to come over and take footage of us. She interviewed Isidro, the girls, and me regarding our experiences as a family. She did a wonderful job in depicting a healthy American family living a full, happy, and, above all, normal lifestyle.

But still, the girls learned early on about people's ignorance regarding disabilities when they saw how others reacted to us because of our physical limitations. There were so many examples of people saying or doing ignorant stuff, such as the time when we were at the register after shopping for groceries and one of the cashiers said to Ariana, "Do you mind helping her out? You are nice for doing that." Ariana was surprised by such a direct and ignorant question. On the way home, Ariana acknowledged the situation and said, "Mom, she was rude for thinking that I take care of you."

We took a vacation at least once a year. We started vacationing when they were two years old and have continued until this day. Both Ariel and Ariana have learned firsthand about the difficulties we face to find suitable access, even with the ADA. During some of our trips, it was challenging for us to find accessible rooms. We sometimes had to change resorts because they didn't have adequate accommodations for us. I am sure that they developed greater patience, though often they voiced anger toward how things are. I am amazed how they've become advocates for accessibility. They are accustomed to reading the fine print to find accessibility features. As I often told them, "Do you see my picture?" They know that handicapped access is always marked with the universal blue wheelchair sign.

Years earlier when the girls were still very little, the first vacation we all took together was to nearby Lake Geneva, Wisconsin. Tom, who owned a time-share, got us a week's stay. We were brave to travel with toddlers, but we also brought along a companion, Reyna's daughter, my niece and goddaughter, Erika. We couldn't do much, but at least the change of scenery was great. Ariana's favorite activity was to play with the garden rocks right outside our condo. We also went on a boat ride which could have ended badly. Isidro was instructed on how to operate the small boat, but as Erika and I were busy getting the girls ready, I overheard when they strongly warned him to "not go beyond the blue flags around the lake." We started our tour, and I was pleased with how Isidro was navigating. This was until I saw him getting too close to the blue flags. I said, "You were told not to go past the blue flags." He said, "Oh, they just say that because they don't want us to see those areas that are probably more beautiful."

Just as he finished responding, he crossed the blue flags. We didn't go too far before the little boat got stuck. He panicked and said, "What should I do?" I said, "I don't know; you were the one who was trained." Clearly concerned, he said, "Weren't you listening? You know I forget things." Irritated, I said, "Well, I told you not to go past the blue flags, but you did." He started to press any button he saw. Sweating, he said, "What should I do?" Since I was the one who'd called to make the boat reservation, I still had the number on my cell phone. I redialed and said, "Hi, we just rented a boat. We are the couple with disabilities. We are stuck and we need help." They asked, "What is your location?" I took a quick look and responded, "We are by a huge bridge," and then gave him the lake's marker. He said to hang tight and they would come to help. It's not like we had any other choice. They pulled us out, but I knew it was futile to tell Isidro "I told you so."

Another two memorable vacations we took when the girls were still too little to remember was going to Kings Island in Ohio, near Cincinnati. This amusement park is a dreamland for toddlers because, like at Disney World, they can see characters that are on their favorite kids' TV shows. The girls were able to take pictures with Dora the Explorer, Blue from *Blue's Clues*, and SpongeBob SquarePants. Even though we couldn't get onto the rides with them, we allowed them to get on rides where we could always see them. They had a great time!

We also went on a cruise to the Bahamas. For this trip, we asked my sister Kika to accompany us. The girls were about three years old, and everyone noticed how cute they were dressed. Some people asked if they were twins, even though they looked so different. Ariana was still tiny while Ariel was much bigger. We always wanted the girls to have the best memories. Perhaps our goal was to compensate for anything that they lacked because of having two parents with disabilities.

CHAPTER 22

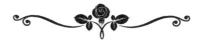

My dad was still missed very much, and we were not prepared for another big loss that would affect the entire family. Not even a year after my dad passed, Kika's only daughter, Jackie, died in September of 2008 at the age of twenty-seven. She'd been diagnosed with lupus in her teen years, but she always gave a good fight. It was devastating for Kika and the entire family to say goodbye to such a loving, beautiful young person. Even my daughters, who were often babysat by Jackie, struggled with this loss. To help them work through their pain, I had Ariel and Ariana write a letter to Jackie. I recorded them as they read their letter. Ariana told me that she was always going to keep a Hannah Montana shirt that Jackie had given her. To this day, Ariana still preserves the shirt with tags and all.

Personally, I really struggled with her death and questioned how God made decisions about who lives and who dies. After I learned about how polio affected me and how I had no medical care, I wondered why God allowed me to live. Jackie, on the other hand, had the best medical care, with the best doctors, yet nothing helped her. I even experienced a form of survivor's guilt. I knew that our conditions were different but still wondered why I was brought back to life. Perhaps this lingering question was my motivation to keep pushing, as if wanting to discover my own purpose.

Equally difficult was knowing how to console Kika. How do you console a grieving mother? Even today, Kika has not found consolation. My mom remained strong to try to help Kika, even when she too was suffering, especially considering she'd just said goodbye not even a year earlier to her husband of fifty-seven years. Kika began to seclude herself and lost her spark for life. Her husband and two sons, Eddie and Netito, did all they could to help her move on. One way that the entire family grieved such a great loss was by participating in the yearly lupus walk in honor of Jackie. They collectively raised money and donated it to the Lupus Foundation to fund more research on better treatment for lupus.

I don't know if the two family losses and my new diagnosis of Post-Polio Syndrome did something to me. But, since the girls no longer needed my physical presence as intensely either, I began to find my own solace behind the computer. After I left campus for the day, I was *done*. I'd worked so hard that, by the time I got home, it was all I could do to get off my chair and sit on my bed. I hid behind the computer doing work, writing, watching novelas, and playing online poker. I found an escape by forming relationships with poker players all over the world. It was a new discovery, and it began to consume my thoughts. I formed fantasies about the people I met, knowing that it was likely I would never meet them. I would stay up late, playing and chatting with these virtual friends.

This newfound diversion took a lot of my time, yet I believed that it was my way to avoid falling into depression. As I was nearing my 50s, many thoughts clouded my mind. I was tired of struggling, and online gaming and relationships served as an escape. I could reinvent myself by being whoever I wanted to be, which often ended up being someone who didn't have a disability. I made friendships with people from Iowa, Maine, Boston, California, South Carolina, and even France. It wasn't until much later that I revealed my disability. I only ended up meeting a couple of those friends face to face. But the time I spent served its purpose when I needed it.

One online friend proved to me that the world is smaller than we think and that we are all interconnected. I had no idea that one of my faculty colleagues, Marianne, was the daughter of a friend I met while playing Texas Hold'em poker. During small talk, I shared that I played online poker as a hobby and diversion. My colleague said, "Oh, my father also plays poker online." I then said, "I play for free chips, so no money is invested." She chimed in, "So does my father. What site do you play on?" I replied, "Pokerstars." Going back and forth, we discovered that her father, Grizzly, was one of my buddies online. That summer, Marianne arranged for me to meet Grizzly when he came down from California to see his family. Indeed, we live in a small world.

Even with this consuming hobby, I continued to work hard. My girls were finishing their primary education. Ariel continued struggling academically, so I pushed her middle school into testing her for learning disabilities. All along I had suspected that there was a reason Ariel had been struggling. When they finally evaluated her, it proved that I had been right from the beginning. She was diagnosed with a learning disability in language. Her IQ proved that she was intelligent, but her processing affected her reading and writing. By the time she entered high school, she qualified for services under the law. She was given an individualized education plan (IEP) that listed her accommodations.

Adolescence is difficult for most, but for Ariel, it was the most challenging time of her life. Besides being diagnosed with a learning disability, she started exhibiting other concerning behaviors. Her doctor referred us to a psychologist who diagnosed Ariel with anxiety. She'd turned fifteen and become defiant. She was a good kid but was resisting what she was feeling. I knew it was difficult for her to deal with the fact that she had disabilities and was also adopted. Her grades began to plummet, and the more she was pushed, the more she resisted. She began to express her feelings when I least expected it. I said, "Ariel, if you get more organized, you wouldn't be so frazzled." And then out of the blue she said, "Mom, I am not wired like you and

Ariana. I don't have your genes." I knew then that her adoption was on her mind. We were in a constant battle. I took her to see a psychologist, and though he didn't help my relationship with her, she did lose a lot of weight on her own. This helped with her feelings about herself.

Ariel was struggling emotionally. The girls were still staying with my mom. I constantly checked in with them to ensure that they still wanted to sleep over there, but they loved being with her. Ariana even slept in the same bed with my mom. But Ariel slept in her own room. My mom kept a close watch, but I noticed that Ariel wanted more freedom. I had refused to get the girls cell phones until they started high school, but now Ariel was constantly on the phone. She was my high drama daughter who got hung up on issues with her friends. She was in her first relationship and kept breaking the phone rules. Plus, I was worried that the relationship was unhealthy because she kept transferring money from her part-time job to her boyfriend. Writing was my best way to communicate with her. Here is the first paragraph of a letter I sent her on October 27, 2016:

A letter from the heart for my daughter Ariel—

Ariel, I love you. You may think I don't understand you, but I do. You are now a young woman, and I want to treat you as one. But I need your help. I want to trust that you will make the right decisions and that you will not be hurt. I want to believe that what I have taught you in life matters to you. I want to protect you from being hurt and don't want any tears to roll down your face. I am strict and I know at times that may seem to be unfair or cruel, but I have such high expectations for you. I am proud of you for who you are, for your strength, your tough personality, and your determination. Sometimes, I want to just hold you and want you to want my advice. I have told you time and time again that NO ONE wants the best for you more than I do.

Her behavior required more focused attention from me, so I began to dedicate more time to her and distance myself from the computer. I felt sad that I'd helped so many students but couldn't help my own daughter. We didn't agree on almost anything. But I finally discovered that the best way for us to communicate was through texting. At least in texts she would share how she felt, though it sometimes hurt. I wanted to convince her to get counseling, but she refused. I still remember one of the most difficult conversations we ever had. Trying to have a positive relationship, I asked, "Ariel, what do you want for Christmas this year?" I was not prepared for her answer when she said, "I want to meet my birth mother." I don't know how I found the words but said, "If that is what you want, I can see if I can help you. Remember, it's not all up to us. She has to want it too." Though it was a difficult conversation, I think it was the best. She learned that I would be her support no matter what.

Work was a good distraction from home challenges. I would drive the girls to school and then go to work. At work, I was developing closer relationships with students, especially the Latino students. A few of them even called me their Harper mom. I was awarded for this by winning the "Extra Five Minute" award which was given to a faculty member who went above and beyond to support students. I was totally surprised about this award. When the Provost called and said she wanted to meet with me, I worried that it was for a student issue. Instead, she came to notify me that students had nominated me to get this award.

Students have always touched my life. The three students who called me Harper mom will always be special to me. First, Gaby, who struggles with learning disabilities, connected with me because I always helped her academically and personally. She lacked self-confidence but was a very hard-working student. Despite her difficulties, she completed her Associates of Applied Science in Human Services. In addition, she was an ADS student aide, so when a position opened, she applied and was hired. I was proud of her success and especially loved seeing her in the office every day. Regardless of what happens, Gaby will be in my life.

Juan is my second Harper child. Besides having a learning disability, he also has a physical disability because of gun violence. He was very angry and had not come to terms with his new disability and becoming a wheelchair user. Because of this, he'd continued his involvement with bad influences and ended up in prison. Throughout his incarceration, I kept in touch with him via letters, reminding him that the college would always be ready for him after his release. After serving his time, he did enroll at Harper again and was a new man with a deep desire to prosper. He worked hard in all his classes and he became involved with the Latinos Unidos student club. He went on to transfer to Northern Illinois University where he is currently pursuing his bachelor's degree in business. Juan is special to me and is someone who helped me as much as I hope I helped him. He proved that success belongs to anyone who wants it. I know that anyone can make miracles happen.

My third and youngest Harper daughter is Daisy. Daisy is simply beautiful, inside and out. She has a diagnosed anxiety disorder and comes from a low-income family. She is very intelligent and even with the struggles that no one her age should have, she perseveres. She helps support her family and does it unselfishly. She is one of the most generous and giving people I know. She always showed her deep appreciation with simple, yet meaningful, expressions of love. I still have all her cards and gifts, which I know she wrote and bought with her whole heart. Daisy is also a firm believer in Jesus and knows that He and only He can help us through our hard times. Even with all her responsibilities, she has participated in numerous missionary trips. I admire her for who she is. I would do anything to support her.

These three students are just a few of the many students I met during my work at Harper College. Many have moved on, hopefully to continuing with a successful life. Some I keep in touch with through social media, holiday cards, and email. Others, like my three Harper children, will always be special to me. They helped me probably more than I helped them. They are my constant reminders of why God wanted me to have another chance and why I woke up from my polio coma. They are beautiful rose gardens that grew from my many years of suffering and tears.

My disability never stopped me from living life to the fullest or helping my own daughters have many different experiences. Once they grew up, we started to vacation to locations farther away. Most often we would take road trips so that we knew we would have reliable, accessible transportation. We've driven as far as Miami, Florida; Canada; and South Padre Island, Texas. We have been to Disney World in Orlando three times—the first time when the girls were eleven, the second when they were thirteen, and most recently when they were adults over eighteen. Instead of a quinceañera, the traditional Mexican celebration held when turning fifteen, we went to Hawaii. We went on another cruise to Belize and Honduras as their high school graduation gift. We have formed long-lasting memories. Perhaps because of my own childhood when I was never able to take a vacation, I have put a high priority on our need to take these trips.

I constantly strived to serve my students in the best way possible. As a full professor, I saw it as my responsibility to always put students first. I dedicated my career to being the voice for those who are marginalized, which includes students with disabilities and the large, growing number of Latino students. The college's president appointed me to be on a task force to discuss diversity and inclusion issues on campus. It was important for me to strive to make Harper a better, more welcoming college for diverse students. In addition, I had the opportunity to work closely with one of my favorite friends, Juanita.

In 2017, I was observing a new need on campus as students with more complex disabilities began enrolling in larger numbers. As I worked more closely with faculty, I recognized that they were struggling to know how to best serve their students with disabilities. I decided to apply for another sabbatical leave. The focus of this leave would be to create material to help faculty know how to best accommodate and support students. My application was approved, so I spent the semester doing research, contacting past students, and writing.

During the spring break of my sabbatical, we went on vacation to South Padre Island, which is near the Mexico border. We wanted to try to arrange for Ariel to meet her birth mom. Unfortunately, Kika's friend said that her birth mom didn't want to meet her. I was concerned that this would be devastating for Ariel. After finding out the news, I talked to Ariel and said, "Ariel, you will not be able to meet your birth mom." Ariel asked why. I said, "She does not want a meeting. Please know that this is not about you; it's about her not being ready." I explained that we didn't know the circumstances under which she was adopted and said her birth mom must have her reasons. I then said, "If you want, we can still go to Mexico so you can see where you were born." She thought for a second and responded, "No, it's OK." She didn't give a reason, but I figured it might have been because immigration was a hot topic at the time and she could have had anxiety about crossing the border.

When the weather started getting better, I would sit outside to write my project. I loved observing my mom and how hard she worked in the garden. I did notice that, in the blink of an eye, she had aged. She was taking more medications for her blood pressure, and her walking appeared more labored. Many people told me that, after my dad's death, she continued living only because she had my girls. Even with her aging, she still put everyone else first. If I needed help with anything, she would be the first person I could count on. If one of my cats ran out, I'd call her on speed dial to catch it. Even when my van got stuck in the snow in the back alley the previous winter, I called her. I felt guilty, but before I knew it, she was out there with a broom and a plastic pumpkin filled with salt to help me. As I watched her, I felt so honored to be her daughter. I thought to myself, *I hope to be even ten percent of the woman she is.*

Expressing my love for her in words was not something I practiced. However, I do hope that I showed her how much I loved her. I had paid her weekly for caring for my girls, then just kept on paying her even after they grew up. She felt bad and often tried to return the money to me, but I said, "This is your retirement pension payment." However, she tried to continue earning the money. She had a key to my house, so often I would notice that she had taken my trash out. She also bought all the gardening supplies and left my yard looking splendid. I could never repay her for all she did for me.

My sabbatical leave resulted in my developing a course for faculty with tips and suggestions for how best to accommodate and support students with the ten most common types of disabilities. I taught the course for the first time in the Fall of 2018, and through that, I got to know faculty in a whole different capacity. The class filled up and the faculty members were engaged completely. I developed close friendships with several of the faculty members, including one who became my honorary Latina friend. Kathleen, an ESL faculty member with a heart of gold, was fluent in Spanish, and the more I got to know her, the more I felt blessed to have her as a friend. And there was also Anne, whom I worked with for so many years since she was a counselor, but who I really got to know because of the class. She provided support during the most difficult times for me.

Positive friendships also resulted from my involvement with Diverse Relationships Engaged in Affirming Multiculturalism (DREAM). The DREAM association aimed at supporting faculty and staff of color while employed at Harper. Veronica, who is now one of my dear friends, was the DREAM chair. I got to know her after she returned from a medical leave. I admired Veronica because, even with her health challenges, she always remained positive. Gerardo, a new Spanish faculty member whom I mentored through DREAM, became one of my dearest friends in a short time. I felt comfortable with him the moment I met him. His sense of humor brightened many of my days.

ADS had experienced many changes as a department, but the friendships I maintained outside the office reinforced my energy and dedication to making Harper a welcoming college. I enjoyed collaborating with my colleagues through DREAM and through a practice community that Kathleen and I had started to help faculty in developing relationships with their students. These friends became my support network not only professionally but also personally. We always had good laughs together and were comfortable just being ourselves. I know that they didn't care about my disability. They would tease me because I was over-ambitious and always got things done in half the time I told them I would need.

Around this time, I started to contemplate retirement. Because of my Post-Polio Syndrome, I was feeling extreme fatigue. I was also diagnosed with type 2 diabetes, among other health conditions. Turning fifty didn't sit well with me. Aging and disability do not get along! I had the desire to work on other projects without the commitment of having to go in to work every day. Additionally, I felt that God was sending me messages, letting me know that my time at Harper was over. I knew I had to figure out the best timing for my retirement but hoped it would come soon because I was struggling to keep my motivation.

Several life-changing events happened in 2018 that made things worse for me. First, because of Ariel's desire to grow up fast, not long after turning eighteen, she decided to move out with a boyfriend she had only known for a few months. We were struggling with her maintaining the rules we had for our household and she wanted more freedom. So, in January 2018, she moved out. I was devastated, wondering why I had failed. I reminded Ariel that our home would always be hers. I said, "I will always support your health and your education. We are here whenever you need us." I couldn't do anything to stop her from making this decision. I knew it wasn't the life I wanted for her, but I just hoped that she would find happiness and be well. This changed our lives. Suddenly, we had become a family of three. I made sure that Ariel knew that I loved her and would always welcome her with open arms.

Ariana, however, was following what I envisioned was best for my daughters. She stayed focused in high school and graduated at the top five percent of her class. She decided to attend Harper College to take advantage of the free tuition benefit I had. Her career goal was to study medicine. However, she recognized that she was an introvert and so probably wouldn't enjoy interacting with patients. She concluded that being a pathologist would be a better fit for her. She entered Harper with a bunch of Advanced Placement credits and was hired by the admissions office as a student aide, which allowed her to work on campus while maintaining a manageable course load. I knew she was in good hands because my best friend at Harper, Juanita, would keep an eye on her.

The most significant reason why 2018 was probably one of the worst years of my life was because on April 19, 2018, my mom left this earth to join my dad in heaven. Her health took a turn for the worse after the summer of 2017. She still had a full summer of gardening, but around her birthday, she started experiencing heart palpitations. The doctors recommended a pacemaker, and she had the procedure done. However, the doctors hadn't counted on the pacemaker causing other heart issues. Blood was now flowing too rapidly into her heart. She needed constant care; she was unable to walk independently because of these health issues. Our family pulled together to determine the best plan of care for her.

Each of my siblings decided to take a day to care for her. I was responsible for making the schedules and resolving any financial issues. At first, my siblings didn't stay the night, so Ariana continued sleeping over as usual. However, when her health began to decline, each brother and sister took a night to stay with her. It was so difficult to see my mom this way. She had been the one who always cared for us, but now she was dependent on others. We had one last Christmas with her in 2017. Per our tradition, we filled her home with the legacy my parents left behind, a huge loving family. We took our last pictures with her. First, all my siblings and I surrounded her as she sat in the middle. Second, she took a picture with her sons-in-law and daughters-in-law, our partners who had grown to love and respect her. Third, she took a picture with her grandchildren, and fourth she took another with her great-grandchildren. By the time of her death, she had twenty-three grandchildren and twenty-two great-grandchildren, with two more on the way.

During the first few months of the new year, my stress levels skyrocketed. I was dealing with the stress of Ariel moving out, my usual work stresses, and my mom's deteriorating health. And then during one of my usual work-from-home days in the first week of April, I took Ariana to school, picked up a coffee, and then came back home again to get to work. I am not certain what happened, or when it happened, but the rest of the day disappeared from my memory. I picked Ariana up from school and said, "How did I get here?" I was not joking. I had no idea what I was doing. I even drove back home without being aware of what I was doing. Everything that was stored in my short-term memory had been erased. Ariana tried to assess what had happened and said, "Mom, did you fall?" As I checked my head, I responded, "I don't think so. But wait, my hair is wet. Did I take a shower?" Ariana figured that if I had fallen, I would still be on the floor because I would have needed help getting up. She was so concerned that she called Isidro and told him, "Something is wrong with mom. She doesn't remember anything." He came home immediately and verified that I was not acting coherently. They took me to Loyola's ER, fearing that I had suffered a stroke. I was admitted and had many tests done. They concluded that I had a rare condition called Transient Global Amnesia. They explained that my brain had shut down and temporarily erased all my short-term memory.

Fortunately, with this condition, the brain rewires itself after several hours and returns to normal. Parts of that day remain a mystery. I was able to trace some of the things I did by looking at my email and reviewing calls I'd made from my cell phone. Apparently, I'd worked hard because I'd even created a PowerPoint for an upcoming presentation. I had made several calls to California, but after analyzing the numbers, it was obvious that I thought I was at my office on campus because all the calls started with an eight, which I have to dial in the office to get an outside number. My mind had given me an eighteen-hour vacation. It is interesting that our minds sometimes protect us when we need it most.

Sadly, even with that temporary amnesia, I still returned to reality and the inevitable. Saying goodbye to the most important person in my life was unbearable. I would visit my mother each night and, even with her failing health, she always showed concern for me. In the winter, my feet get extremely cold, so when I visited her, she would ask for my feet so that she could warm them up with her loving hands. We had many meaningful conversations when I went over to see her. In one of our conversations she said, "I have run out of extensions," referring to the conversation we'd had when Ariana was born. She said, "Your girls are now grown and no longer need me." I quickly responded, "Mom, we all need you." She just smiled and said, "My work is done."

Mom then asked my sister to get her a little tin box she had always used to store valuable documents. My sister and I had no idea what she wanted. She rummaged through the box and took out a worn-out piece of paper. It was obvious that the folded document had been read many times and then folded back up. She handed it to me and said, "Read this." I opened the letter carefully, not wanting to rip it, and I immediately recognized the writing. It was Isidro's handwriting. I read the letter, and the date was before Isidro and I were married. It was surprising for me to know that Isidro had written a letter to my mom before our marriage. In the letter he promised my mom that he loved me and would always protect me. I teared up and said, "I had no idea he had written this to you. He never told me." She said, "This letter is what helped me survive when you moved to Texas." It was apparent that she had read it many times and that she treasured it. When she told me I could keep it, I didn't know that she was starting to say goodbye.

I had another conversation with her about Isidro. She said, "I am so happy you found the perfect partner for your life." I said, "Yes, he is a good man." She said, "When it is time for me to go, I'll be ready because I won't worry about you." I said, "Mom, I still need you and will always need you." She said, "You will be fine without me." I didn't want to fathom the idea that someday she would be gone. However, I understood what she was saying. Though my siblings are all very loving, each of my brothers and sisters had their own family and wouldn't be able to help me like my mom had for so many years. But I had my own family, and my mom recognized that they would be the best support for me.

My mom was very lucid and wise, even with her failing health. She was still aware of everything. It was painful for her to learn that Ariel had moved out with her boyfriend. During one of my visits, she said, "Make sure to help Ariel." I said, "Mom, it was her choice to move out." She said, "I know. But you are her mom and if you don't help her, who will?" I asked, "How can I help her if she doesn't live here anymore?" She said, "Give her the car and help her with anything she needs." When Ariel moved out, I told her that she had to leave the car that we had bought for her. I also told her that I wouldn't help her financially except with her health and education. My mom's love for her family surpassed any boundary, though, so she helped me realize that I should always be supportive to my daughters, regardless of any mistakes they ever make.

Probably the most significant conversation I had with my mom during the last weeks of her life was when she said, "I finally know the answer." Taking her hand, I asked, "Answer about what?" She said, "Since you were born, I looked for an answer of why you got polio." I immediately remembered that we often discussed reasons for why I was chosen to be disabled. In fact, on several occasions she wanted to blame herself, but I would always tell her to stop. I asked, "Why do you think I got polio?" She said, "So you could help so many students with disabilities. You were meant to work with them to inspire them." This was the best explanation I ever received. It had been my destiny to go through so many valleys of tears so that I could be humbled and be the support to other people with disabilities. I wanted to tell her how much I loved her, but as usual, the words didn't come out. I just hugged her.

Two weeks later, my mom was put into hospice care. It was a difficult decision for our family because we knew this meant that there was no hope for her, and the goal was just to keep her comfortable. Every day, a nurse would come to take her vitals. She was hardly eating yet still very aware. I was scheduled to go to a conference; I contemplated canceling my trip but everyone, including the nurse, told me that she might be the same way for weeks. It was hard for me to decide to go, but I felt obligated because the college had already paid my airfare and registration fee. Besides, my mom was stable, or at least I thought.

Juanita and I went to Los Angeles. As soon as I got to the hotel, I called my mom. I didn't know that I was having my last conversation with her. I said, "Hi, mom. How are you?" She said, "I am fine. Did you eat?" I said, "Yes, mom. I am in Los Angeles but will come back in three days. What do you want me to take you?" She said, "Cigarettes." Confused, I said, "Why cigarettes when you don't smoke?" My mother had never smoked in her entire life. She responded, "You are right. I have never been good for even that." On multiple occasions she always felt that she was inferior because she had not done many of the things other women had done. She was so humble for not recognizing that she had been the best daughter, wife, mother, mother-in-law, grandmother, aunt, and human being.

After the call, I was left restless. I called Isidro, who was working from home. He had gone back to school at Harper and received certification as a medical office assistant, so he'd left the business world to start working for a medical insurance company. I said, "I just talked to mom. Please go visit her every day. I am not in peace." He said, "I was planning to do that anyway. Don't worry." I hung up the phone, but something told me that I should not be in California. Although I was physically at the conference, my mind and heart were with my mother.

My mom's health took a turn for the worse. I received a call from her nurse, since I was the contact who had arranged for hospice. She told me that mom was now unresponsive and that they were making her comfortable. There was no way I could continue at the conference. I told Juanita I had to leave immediately but that she should stay. She said, "I will not stay. I will leave with you." We paid an extra fee to switch our flights, and I promised Juanita I would pay her back. She said, "No way. I am leaving because I want to and because I care for you." At the airport, Isidro called and said, "Cuali, your mom is just waiting for you. Are you coming back?" I responded, "Yes. I'm at the airport and will arrive at 7 PM." He said, "Good! Let me know when you get here so I can pick you up."

No flight had been so long, not even the flight to Hawaii. I was desperate to get home. I was feeling awful for having left her. Juanita was like a sister, helping me prepare for the worst day of my life. She tried to calm me down and console me, but I was a complete wreck. When I arrived at the airport, I called Isidro to come pick me up. I said farewell to Juanita and thanked her. I could see her concern for me because she was aware of what I was about to go through. In the minivan, Isidro updated me on my mom. He said, "The whole family is there. They all think she is just waiting for you." By now, I let the floodgates open and began crying.

I went immediately to my mom's house and quickly headed to her bedroom without saying hello to anyone. I cried and asked my mom, "What happened? I left you OK." I grabbed her hand and began to caress her. She was surrounded by family members. Crying I said, "I love you, mom. If you need to go, it is OK. I'll be alright!" She was breathing with difficulty, so my niece Vanessa wet her dry lips with a soaked piece of cotton. I hoped that she was listening to me. I repeated, "Mom. It's OK if you leave to be with dad. I am going to be fine." Vanessa, using her phone, played "Somewhere over the Rainbow" as I continued talking to her. I was thinking to myself, *Why didn't I tell her how much I loved her more often?* I stayed there for a couple of hours, each minute hurting more than the previous. I couldn't handle not seeing her beautiful, loving brown eyes. My sister Tere was going to spend the night. She insisted that we all go home and that she would alert us if there was any change. Although I was extremely tired, I left only because I lived right next door and could rush over at any moment.

I probably slept a couple of hours because I knew difficult days were coming. I got up very early to go see her, but when I was in the bathroom brushing my teeth, my nephew came to say that my mom had died. With a mouth full of toothpaste, I wailed in turmoil. I quickly rinsed my mouth and went over. She looked so peaceful, but I couldn't believe her soul was no longer in her body.

After my dad's death, my mom had arranged to be buried next to him. My older brothers took care of the arrangements; her grandchildren created a video and collected pictures; and I wrote her obituary. It was challenging to write in just a few words all that my mom meant to us. This is the obituary that was published but that doesn't capture all that my mom signified to us:

> Virginia Herrera's job on earth is done! She was called to eternal peace on April 19, 2018. She was an extraordinary human being, a devoted daughter of the late Petra and Consolación Diaz, a loving wife of the late Eulalio Herrera, mother of Bella (Baltazar) Corral, Angelita (Humberto) Olivarez, Tere (Ismael) Navar, Kika (Ernesto) Silva, Mon (Edilia) Herrera, Reyna (Lencho) Duarte, Lalo (Irene) Herrera, Cuali (Isidro) Herrera, and Rique (Betty) Herrera, and grandmother to 23 grandchildren, great-grandmother to 22 with 2 on the way. Sister to 5 siblings, and aunt to many. Virginia was a servant by nature, caring for her family, her greatest treasure. She tended to her garden full of flowers with the same devotion to and love as she tended to the needs of everyone she encountered. She will never be forgotten. Family and friends are to gather for the Visitation Friday, April 20, 2018 from 3:00 PM–9:00 PM

at Russo's Hillside Chapels, 4500 Roosevelt Road, Hillside, Illinois 60162 (located between Mannheim and Wolf Road). Funeral Saturday, April 21, 2018, from Russo's Hillside Chapels at 8:30 AM, proceeding to the Shrine of Our Lady at St. Charles Borromeo Catholic Church, 1637 N 37th Avenue, Melrose Park, Illinois 60160. Mass of Christian Burial celebrated promptly at 10:00 AM. Interment at Mount Emblem Cemetery at 520 E. Grand Avenue, Elmhurst, Illinois 60126.

The wake was overcrowded with people who came to give their regards to a woman who had touched them in one way or another. I don't think I had ever seen so many people. I went through the wake and funeral numb. It was surreal, as if I were living in a horrible nightmare. Father Luis, my friend from DePaul who had celebrated my parents' fiftieth wedding anniversary, was now officiating my mom's funeral eighteen years later. After the Mass, the procession to the cemetery was miles long. We even made a special point to drive by their small Franklin Park home that had welcomed so many people. Anyone would have thought that a celebrity had died. However, it was just my mom, a simple, humble woman who had dignified the world with her existence.

The burial was more difficult than I had anticipated. It's as if I'd finally woken up from my daze and realized what was really happening. As soon as I got out of the minivan and saw the crowd surrounding the coffin, I lost it. I screamed, "Please don't put her in there!" I was unable to breathe and would have literally gotten up to stop them. She was so beautiful in the golden dress that she had last worn to celebrate fifty years of happiness with my dad. It was as if all our tears and suffering had washed away her wrinkles, making her look angelic. It finally hit me that this was it. I would no longer see her. I would no longer be able to be totally myself and be totally understood. How would I live without her? She had been the wind beneath my wings. All that I was I owed to her. I really didn't know how I would continue living.

According to our culture and Catholic customs, we celebrated a novena in her name. For nine days after her burial, we all met in her house. We set an altar with the many beautiful flowers and plants we had received. My sisters Bella and Angelita lead the prayer. Each night we filled every room in the house until it was standing room only. We took turns passing food around at the conclusion of the rosary. All my nieces and nephews worked in unison as if we had hired them to be servers. I felt proud that everyone was able to see the remarkable woman I knew and adored. It was extremely difficult to get through the entire novena, but I was content. I hoped she was watching from heaven and would finally realize that she wasn't as insignificant as she had often felt throughout her life.

CHAPTER 23

After my mom's passing, I had many dark moments. I missed her so much! As I left for work in the morning, I missed seeing her laboring in her garden or her offering me a fresh cup of arroz con leche. How I wish I had accepted every cup she'd offered. At home when I couldn't reach something, I almost dialed her number so that she could run over to get me what I needed. When the cat ran out, I thought of her because she would so often come to the rescue. But now she was gone and couldn't help me. I knew my brothers and sisters and the entire family missed her, but I not only missed her, I *needed* her. This realization made me feel guilty for a long time. I felt that all I brought to her was heartache. She had suffered so much because of me. I hated to think about how much she had cried because of the polio and its aftermath. She had brought me back to life, but now I had to learn how to live without her.

As I tended to do, I numbed myself by pushing forward. My group of friends sustained me and brought smiles to me at work. The whole family supported one other, especially through the process of getting her home ready to sell. We cleared everything out, many of us taking pictures and other items that were significant to us. Her broken-down toaster oven in which she had cooked endless amounts of pizza, her many flowerpots and vases, and her personal belongings all found homes in our families. She was such a minimalist and was content with what she had. We found crates full of unopened, unused gifts we had given her over the years. The only thing that I wanted to make sure I had was her bed where Ariana had slept with her for so many years. Everyone agreed that the bed belonged to Ariana. I remember my oldest brother telling Ariana, "You deserve this bed. Mom lived so many more years because of you and Ariel."

We sold the house, and my oldest brother Mon and my oldest sister Bella equally divided our inheritance. I put the money in the bank, painfully remembering all the sacrifices my parents had made to leave us something after their deaths. What they didn't know is that they had already left us the best inheritance ever—our love for each other and our unity. Though my mom was the conduit for keeping us all united, we all vowed that we would continue to be unified and to look out for each other. This is a promise that I have no doubt we will keep. My parents planted a good harvest and would now be happy observing what they sowed.

Since her death, I haven't been the same. I felt an important piece of me was missing. My daughters were now finding their own paths. My relationship with Ariel improved because I listened to my mother's advice to always be there to support her. She even returned home to her family. Ariana was prospering with her goals, earning a lot of scholarships and recognition for her hard work. Isidro continued to be my partner who I could always depend on. At work I was being successful and getting recognition from the campus. I was still touching students' lives as best I knew how. But things were not the same.

Even despite what was happening with me emotionally with the loss of my mom, a group of faculty members led by Marianne and Veronica nominated me for the 2019 Distinguished Faculty Award. This is the highest recognition bestowed annually to a deserving faculty member. It was very humbling when I was selected. In addition to a monetary award, I was invited to speak to an audience during Harper's convocation. When I was notified, the only person I thought about was my mom. She had always been in the shadows cheering for me. Each accomplishment I had ever received was because of her. From that awful time of contracting polio to the time when I had my own family, she was always there. I decided to dedicate my speech to her. The audience was touched, evidenced by a standing ovation, because I spoke from my heart. Here is the speech I gave:

Good evening, everyone.

I am honored to have been selected as this year's distinguished faculty. I want to thank the Motorola Solutions Foundation for this Endowed Award for Teaching Excellence, the faculty who nominated me for this recognition, my Student Development Division who supported my nomination, and the award selection committee for selecting me for this prestigious award.

Abraham Lincoln once said, "All that I am or hope to be, I owe to my angel Mother." This is indeed true for me. You see, to this day, my mother continues to be the wind beneath my wings even though she left this earth a year ago in April. No one would have imagined that I, a low-income Latina who was diagnosed with polio at the age of nine months in Mexico and crawled around until coming to the United States, would someday be here accepting such a distinctive honor. My mom often wondered why God chose me to acquire this disease when her other eight children were spared. Throughout my life, she often posed that same question, often seeking an answer for the cause of my condition that left me unable to walk. I believe that it was my disability and my parents' hope that motivated them to come to the United States for a better life when I was seven years old.

Even after I became independent by adjusting to my disability, pursued the American dream through an education, and got married and formed my own family, she always had that question. It wasn't until a couple of weeks before passing away in April of 2018 that she told me that she finally found the answer. In her frail voice, she told me that she discovered that I had to have a disability so that I could motivate and support students with disabilities in working hard to find their own path.

My mom was one of the wisest women I will ever know. She pointed out the obvious. She helped me realize that my work at Harper was not just a job, or even a career. My work at Harper has been my life's purpose and my passion. I am very fortunate to have the certainty of knowing why I was put on this earth.

I am extremely blessed that my path led me to Harper College in August of 1991. Harper has offered me many opportunities to grow professionally and most importantly personally. Besides having positive mentors, I have worked with countless students with varying disabilities, each helping me to develop and grow professionally and each teaching me a lesson that made me the person I am today. I have grown in my faith and my philosophy of education has become even more solidified. Now I am certain that every person, every student, regardless of their diversity, is valuable, has potential, and has a purpose.

I am beyond grateful for life for allowing me to work at Harper where I've had the privilege of working with many dedicated faculty and staff. Whether it is to work on a project or program, be on a committee, or to consult about a student, I discovered that there are many distinguished faculty and staff here at Harper who are equally invested in giving students the hope they need to succeed in life. Many of these employees are no longer just coworkers but have become my dearest friends and members of my Harper family. Colleagues, my only wish for you is that you continue to use the tremendous power you have as educators to help students achieve their dreams regardless of their abilities, disabilities, or other forms of diversity.

To all the students being recognized this evening and even to those who weren't, I want you to know that we believe in YOU. You will find your own path that will lead you to discover your own purpose, even if it is later in life like I did. Work hard, believe in your own potential, dream high, and above all, make your mark with respect and kindness. For it is through the impact you have on others that you will truly be successful. Dream the impossible, arm yourself with the support of others, and believe me, the impossible will someday become a reality.

Lastly, to my husband, my two beautiful daughters, and my eight siblings and their families, I want you to know that you are the world to me. I appreciate you for always being present and cheering for me, especially when I doubted my ability to continue. Your unconditional love has never gone unnoticed.

My dear mother in heaven, you never gave up on me, even when you were told that my future didn't look promising, I dedicate this recognition to you! All that I am, and all that I still hope to be, I owe it to you.

Thank you!

Additionally, I was humbled once again when I was nominated and selected to be on the National Disability Mentoring Coalition Hall of Fame. Every year, individuals are honored for making a difference through mentorship in the lives of people with disabilities. I had no idea that I had been nominated by my first Harper daughter, Gaby. It is a recognition that I am grateful to have received because I always strived to pay forward the mentoring that I received through my life's journey.

These recognitions were a culminating result of all the hard work I had done. Somehow, I sensed that my time at Harper was concluding, but I also knew that if I retired when I was first eligible, I would be financially penalized. At night, I struggled with deciding on what was next for me. I was not getting much sleep, and my health was impacted by my grief. I realized that I never really allowed myself to mourn the loss of the most significant person in my life.

One restless night, I got up and went into my yard and looked across the fence to the house that used to be my mom's. I looked up to the sky and spoke to my mom. I said, "Mom, I don't know what to do. I am so tired of the fight. If I decide to retire, I will lose a lot of money." My mom responded, not with words but with memories. I remembered that she once had said that decisions based on money are not good. I then continued my conversation, looking up to the sky once again. I said, "Mom, I don't want to feel like I am quitting.

You taught me to never give up." Again, without words, I felt my mom's response. It's as if she said, "You have already surpassed any expectations. You are not quitting. You are just going to reinvent yourself." I had not dreamt of my mom or seen any signs since her death as my brothers and sisters said they did. But that night, my mom supported me like she always had. I went to bed and slept peacefully for a few hours.

After consulting with my doctors and my family, I decided that I would give myself time to focus on myself and my emotional and physical wellness. I requested a medical leave beginning in mid-November, a year and a half after my mom left this earth. I wasn't sure if I would retire at the end of the school year, but I knew I wanted to decide by March. During my medical leave, my daughter suggested that writing a book and dedicating it to my mom might be good therapy for me to help me resolve so many painful memories I had. For her young age, Ariana is so wise. It is no wonder that when she was little and I held her tight I said, "You are a piece of heaven in my arms." Even though I don't hold her in my arms anymore like I did when she was a child, I told Ariana after my mom's passing, "You are a piece of my mom." That to me was a piece of heaven.

God willing, in my future, I will have many reasons to celebrate. I am sure that Ariel will find her way with a job that she loves, and Ariana will finish her studies in something related to the sciences and then will find a good job. Isidro will continue being my faithful companion and I will be his. We will celebrate many wedding anniversaries following the example of my parents, for their values are also part of my inheritance. Without a doubt, I will continue to impact lives in one way or another. God is good!

I retired from my job at the age of fifty-five. I was so scared! I wondered, *What will protect me from my ever-present self-doubt?* I had no idea that writing this memoir would be so therapeutic. I was surprised to remember so many parts of my life. As I wrote and relieved the difficult moments, I cried, but I also celebrated. I'm here. I beat my obstacles. I did it because of God's eternal love and his guidance in finding my life purpose. I don't know what the future has in store for me, but I'm sure I'm ready. My life has been so meaningful and all the tears that I cried served to make me the woman I am today. Yes, there were many valleys of tears; everyone has them. But I conquered, and God rewarded me every day with happy moments with my beautiful family and many friends. I know I did the best I could because my parents taught me to persevere through difficult times in life. I just hope my mom looks down at me and recognizes that the valley of tears she lived on earth got her to the most beautiful garden in heaven.

9 781736 338865